Oxford Case Histories in Obstetric Medicine

T0177537

Oxford Case Histories

Series Editors:
Sarah Pendlebury and Peter Rothwell

Published:
Anaesthesia (Jon McCormack, Keith Kelly)

Cardiology (Rajkumar Rajendram, Javed Ehtisham, Colin Forfar)

Gastroenterology and Hepatology (Alissa J. Walsh, Otto C. Buchel, Jane Collier, Simon P.L. Travis)

General Surgery (Judith E. Ritchie, K. Raj Prasad)

Geriatric Medicine (Sanja Thompson, Nicola Lovett, John Grimley Evans, Sarah Pendlebury)

Infectious Diseases and Microbiology (Hilary Humphreys, William Irving, Bridget Atkins, Andrew Woodhouse)

Lung Cancer (Himender K. Makker, Adam Ainley, Sanjay Popat, Julian Singer, Martin Hayward, Antke Hagena)

Neurosurgery (Harutomo Hasegawa, Matthew Crocker, Pawan Singh Minhas)

Obstetric Medicine (Charlotte Frise, Krupa Bhalsod, Rebecca Scott, Harry Gibson)

Oncology (Thankamma Ajithkumar, Adrian Harnett, Tom Roques)

Respiratory Medicine (John Stradling, Andrew Stanton, Najib M. Rahman, Annabel H. Nickol, Helen E. Davies)

Rheumatology (Joel David, Anne Miller, Anushka Soni, Lyn Williamson)

Sleep Medicine (Himender Makker, Matthew Walker, Hugh Selsick, Bhik Kotecha, Ama Johal)

TIA and Stroke (Sarah T. Pendlebury, Ursula G. Schulz, Aneil Malhotra, Peter M. Rothwell)

Oxford Case Histories in Obstetric Medicine

Charlotte Frise

Consultant Obstetric Physician, Oxford University Hospitals
NHS Foundation Trust, Oxford and Imperial College
Healthcare NHS Trust, London, UK

Krupa Bhalsod

Specialist Registrar in Acute Medicine, West Middlesex
University Hospital, Chelsea and Westminster Hospital NHS
Trust, London, UK

Rebecca Scott

Consultant Obstetric Physician, Diabetologist, and
Endocrinologist, Chelsea and Westminster Hospital,
London, UK

Harry Gibson

Consultant in Obstetrics and Gynaecology, Whittington
Health NHS Trust, London, UK

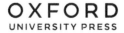

OXFORD
UNIVERSITY PRESS

OXFORD
UNIVERSITY PRESS

Great Clarendon Street, Oxford, OX2 6DP,
United Kingdom

Oxford University Press is a department of the University of Oxford.
It furthers the University's objective of excellence in research, scholarship,
and education by publishing worldwide. Oxford is a registered trade mark of
Oxford University Press in the UK and in certain other countries

First Edition published in 2023

Published in the United States of America by Oxford University Press
198 Madison Avenue, New York, NY 10016, United States of America

British Library Cataloguing in Publication Data
Data available

Library of Congress Control Number: 2022946402

ISBN 978–0–19–284589–4

DOI: 10.1093/med/9780192845894.001.0001

Printed in the UK by
Ashford Colour Press Ltd, Gosport, Hampshire

Dedications

To all those who share our passion for improving outcomes in medically complicated pregnancies

Acknowledgements

Firstly I would like to acknowledge my co-authors, who contributed to this book with energy and enthusiasm despite the massive pressures of working clinically during the pandemic and simultaneously keeping life going at home with their families. We are very grateful for the help and guidance provided by Caroline, Sylvia and their team at OUP which resulted in such a smooth and swift publishing experience.

Finally, I must thank Matt, Emilia, Alexander, Oliver and Theo for their unfailing support and patience whilst I undertook another book!

CF

Thank you to those who have helped me, and continue to help me, on my obstetric medicine journey. Thank you also to Ayana Jasmine, Shreya Radha, Kiyara Neya and Alkesh who fill my life with joy.

KB

Thank you to Professor David Williams for his wisdom and encouragement as a friend and mentor, Professor Cathy Nelson-Piercy for inspiring me to work in this field, and Pete, Martha and Edward for their patience whilst I have contributed to this book.

RS

Thank you to Amma, Cathy and Richard for inspiring me; to Hannah, Kit, Barnaby and Laurie for distracting me.

HG

A note from the series editors

Case histories have always had an important role in medical education, but most published material has been directed at undergraduates or residents. The *Oxford Case Histories* series aims to provide more complex case-based learning for clinicians in specialist training and consultants, with a view to aiding preparation for entry- and exit-level specialty examinations or revalidation.

Each case book follows the same format with approximately 50 cases, each comprising a brief clinical history and investigations, followed by questions on differential diagnosis and management, and detailed answers with discussion.

At the end of each book, cases are listed by mode of presentation, aetiology, and diagnosis. We are grateful to our colleagues in the various medical specialties for their enthusiasm and hard work in making the series possible.

Sarah Pendlebury and Peter Rothwell

Contents

Abbreviations

ABCDE	Airway, Breathing, Circulation, Disability, Exposure
ABG	arterial blood gas
ACE	angiotensin-converting-enzyme
ACR	albumin:creatinine ratio
ACR	American College of Rheumatology
ADH	antidiuretic hormone
AFE	amniotic fluid embolism
AFLP	acute fatty liver of pregnancy
ALP	alkaline phosphatase
ALS	advanced life support
ALT	alanine aminotransferase
ANA	antinuclear antibody
ANCA	anti-nuclear cytoplasmic antibodies
APTT	activated partial thromboplastin time
ASD	atrial septal defect
AST	aspartate aminotransferase
ATA	American Thyroid Association
AV	atrioventricular
AVNRT	AV-nodal re-entrant tachycardia
AVRT	AV-re-entrant tachycardia
BCG	Bacille Calmette-Guerin
bDMARD	biological disease-modifying anti-rheumatic drug
BMI	Body mass index
BNP	brain natriuretic peptide
BP	blood pressure
bpm	beats per minute
cART	combination antiretroviral therapy
CF	cystic fibrosis
CFRD	cystic fibrosis-related diabetes
CFTR	cystic fibrosis transmembrane conductance regulator
CFU	colony forming unit
CGM	continuous glucose monitoring
CK	creatine kinase
CKD	chronic kidney disease
CMV	cytomegalovirus
CPAP	continuous positive airway pressure
CRP	C-reactive protein
CSF	cerebrospinal fluid
CSII	continuous subcutaneous insulin infusion
CT	computerized tomography
CTA	CT angiogram
CTG	cardiotocography
CTPA	computerized tomography pulmonary angiography
CVS	chorionic villus sampling
CXR	chest X-ray
DCDA	dichorionic diamniotic
DCM	dilated cardiomyopathy
DDP	dipeptidyl peptidase
DIC	disseminated intravascular coagulation
DKA	diabetic ketoacidosis
DOAC	direct oral anticoagulant
dsDNA	double stranded DNA
DVT	deep vein thrombosis
EBV	Epstein–Barr virus
EC	epirubicin and cyclophosphamide
ECG	electrocardiogram
ENA	extractable nuclear antigen
ERCP	endoscopic retrograde cholangiopancreatography
ESR	erythrocyte sedimentation rate
EULAR	European League against Rheumatism

FAST	Focused Assessment with Sonography in Trauma	IVC	inferior vena cava
		IVF	*in-vitro* fertilization
FBC	full blood count	IVIG	intravenous immunoglobulin
FeNO	fractional exhaled nitric oxide	JC	John Cunningham (virus)
FEV1	forced expiratory volume in 1 second	JVP	jugular venous pressure
		L	litre
FSH	follicle stimulating hormone	L-CHAD	long-chain-3-hydroxyacyl-CoA dehydrogenase
fT3	free triiodothyronine		
fT4	free thyroxine	LDH	lactate dehydrogenase
FVC	forced vital capacity	LFT	liver function test
FVS	fetal varicella syndrome	LGA	large for gestational age
g	grams	LH	luteinizing hormone
GAS	Group A beta-haemolytic streptococcus	LKM	liver-kidney-microsome
		LMWH	low molecular weight heparin
GCS	Glasgow coma scale	LV	left ventricle
G-CSF	granulocyte colony-stimulating factor	MAHA	microangiopathic haemolytic anaemia
GFR	glomerular filtration rate	MC&S	microscopy, culture, and sensitivity
GGT	gamma-glutamyl transpeptidase		
		MCV	mean corpuscular volume
GLP	glucagon-like peptide	MDT	multidisciplinary team
GP	general practitioner	MERS	Middle Eastern respiratory syndrome
Hb	haemoglobin		
HCG	human chorionic gonadotropin	mg	milligram
HDU	High Dependency Unit	mGy	milligray
HELLP	haemolysis, elevated liver enzymes, low platelet count	MHRA	Medicines and Healthcare product Regulatory Agency
HEV	hepatitis E	ml	millilitre
HG	hyperemesis gravidarum	MMA	methylmalonic acid
HIV	human immunodeficiency virus	MR	magnetic resonance
		MRCP	magnetic resonance cholangiopancreatography
hr	hour		
HSV	herpes simplex virus	MRI	magnetic resonance imaging
HUS	haemolytic uraemic syndrome	MS	multiple sclerosis
IBD	inflammatory bowel disease	NAFLD	non-alcoholic fatty liver disease
ICP	intrahepatic cholestasis of pregnancy	NICE	National Institute for Health and Care Excellence
Ig	immunoglobulin		
IM	intramuscular	NSAID	non-steroidal anti-inflammatory drug
INR	international normalized ratio		
ITP	immune thrombocytopenia	OHSS	ovarian hyperstimulation syndrome
ITU	Intensive Therapy Unit		
		OSA	obstructive sleep apnoea
IV	intravenous	PCR	polymerase chain reaction

PCR	protein:creatinine ratio	SSRI	selective serotonin reuptake inhibitors
PE	pulmonary embolism		
PEP	polymorphic eruption of pregnancy	SUDEP	sudden unexpected death in epilepsy
PET	positron emission tomography	TB	tuberculosis
PG	pemphigoid gestationis	TIA	transient ischaemic attack
PGP	pelvic girdle pain	TMA	thrombotic microangiopathy
PLGF	placental growth factor	TnI	troponin I
PPCM	peripartum cardiomyopathy	TPO	thyroid peroxidase
PRES	posterior reversible encephalopathy syndrome	TSH	thyroid stimulating hormone
		TTP	thrombotic thrombocytopenic purpura
PT	prothrombin time		
PUPPP	pruritic urticarial papules and plaques of pregnancy	UDCA	ursodeoxycholic acid
		US	ultrasound
PUQE	Pregnancy-Unique Quantification of Emesis	UTI	urinary tract infection
		VBAC	vaginal birth after caesarean
RCOG	Royal College of Obstetricians and Gynaecologists	VQ	ventilation/perfusion
		VRIII	variable rate intravenous insulin infusion
RNP	ribonucleoprotein		
SARS	severe acute respiratory syndrome	VTE	venous thromboembolism
		VWF	von Willebrand factor
SCD	sickle cell disease	VZIG	varicella zoster immunoglobulin
SGLT	sodium-glucose co-transporter		
SLE	systemic lupus erythematosus	VZV	varicella-zoster virus
SMA	smooth muscle antibody	WCC	white cell count
SPD	symphysis pubis dysfunction	WHO	World Health Organization

Normal Ranges

These reference ranges apply to the cases within this book. They are for illustration only and should not be used to inform clinical care.

Laboratory Test	Unit	Normal range in pregnancy
Haemoglobin	g/L	Over 110 g/L (first trimester) Over 105 g/L (second and third trimester)
White cell count	×10⁹ cells/L	4.2–11.2
Neutrophil	×10⁹ cells/L	2.0–7.1
Lymphocyte	×10⁹ cells/L	1.1–3.6
Platelets	×10⁹ cells/L	135–400
Sodium	mmol/L	132–142
Potassium	mmol/L	3.5–5.3
Urea	mmol/L	2.5–7.8
Creatinine	µmol/L	< 70
Bilirubin	µmol/L	0–21
Alanine aminotransferase	iu/L	0–34
Alkaline phosphatase	iu/L	230
Albumin	g/L	35–50
Adjusted calcium	mmol/L	2.20–2.60
C-reactive protein	mg/L	0–5
Lactate	mmol/L	0.60–2.50
Lactate dehydrogenase	iu/L	125–243
Ketones	mmol/L	< 0.6
Glucose	mmol/L	3.6–8.0
Glycated haemoglobin (HbA1c)	mmol/mol	< 42
Urate	µmol/L	140–360 (gestation dependent)
Brain natriuretic peptide (BNP)	ng/L	< 155
Creatine kinase	iu/L	40–320

Laboratory Test	Unit	Normal range in pregnancy
Troponin I	ng/L	0–15
Thyroid-stimulating hormone	mU/L	0.3–4.0*
Free triiodothyronine	pmol/L	2.4–6.0
Free thyroxine	pmol/L	8–23*
Vitamin B12	ng/L	160–800
Folate	μg/L	> 2.7
Ferritin	μg/L	> 30
Serum iron	μmol/L	11–30
Transferrin saturation	%	16–50
Transferrin	g/L	1.0–3.6
Bile acids	μmol/L	0–14
pH		7.35–7.45
PaO$_2$	kPa	10.5–13.5
PaCO$_2$	kPa	3.9–5.0
Bicarbonate	mmol/L	20
Base excess	mEq/L	2–3
Chloride	mmol/L	98–106
Prothrombin time	seconds	12.8–17.4
Activated partial thromboplastin time	seconds	25.0–35/0
Fibrinogen	g/L	1.90–4.30
D-Dimer	μg/L	Not clarified
International Normalised Ratio		< 1.2
Urine protein:creatinine ratio	mg/mmol	< 30

*For the purposes of this book, a single reference range is used here. We advise the use of local trimester-specific reference ranges in clinical practice.

Case 1

A 23-year-old woman in her first pregnancy presented at 32 weeks of gestation with a 1-day history of progressively worsening, constant, lower thoracic and upper lumbar back pain. There was no history of trauma or heavy lifting, and no symptoms of urinary retention, faecal incontinence, or neurological symptoms in the lower limbs. Her pregnancy had been uncomplicated prior to this. At booking her BMI was normal and her BP was 95/70 mmHg. She had a past medical history of hypermobility. Her family history included hypertension in her father, and her sister had a history of spontaneous bowel perforation. She was a non-smoker.

Initial assessment

General inspection:	Unwell and in pain
Heart rate:	115 bpm
Blood pressure:	130/80 mmHg
Respiratory rate:	25 breaths/min
Temperature:	37.0 °C
Oxygen saturations:	99% on room air
Urinalysis:	No protein

Examination

Cardiovascular:	Normal heart sounds, no murmurs
Respiratory:	Normal breath sounds
Abdomen:	Soft abdomen, non-tender gravid uterus
Back:	No tenderness over vertebrae
Cervix:	Os closed, no sign of rupture of membranes

Bloods

See Table 1.1.

Table 1.1 Admission bloods

Haemoglobin	110 g/L
WCC	13.7×10^9/L
Platelets	190×10^9/L
Sodium	136 mmol/L
Potassium	4.0 mmol/L
Urea	7.1 mmol/L
Creatinine	80 µmol/L
Bilirubin	8 µmol/L
ALT	20 iU/L
Albumin	28 g/L
CRP	10 mg/L
Amylase	200 U/L
Urate	100 µmol/L

Abdominal ultrasound was performed which showed no abnormality. Over the next 24 hours, she deteriorated with worsening back pain and a reduction in urine output. Her blood pressure was 180/95 mmHg and her heart rate was 130 bpm. She remained afebrile. She was transferred to the High Dependency Unit for monitoring. Repeat bloods are shown in Table 1.2.

Table 1.2 Repeat bloods

Haemoglobin	70 g/L
WCC	18.2×10^9/L
Platelets	185×10^9/L
Urea	11.1 mmol/L
Creatinine	286 µmol/L

Questions

1. What are the potential causes of her presenting symptoms?
2. Why is this diagnosis more common in pregnancy?
3. What investigations would you arrange?
4. How would you manage this condition?
5. What underlying genetic diagnoses must be considered?

Answers

1. What are the potential causes of her presenting symptoms?

Aortic dissection is the most likely diagnosis. It can present with a variety of symptoms, depending on the location and extent of the dissection. Stanford type A aortic dissections are those that involve the ascending aorta (and may also involve the aortic arch or descending aorta) and all others are classified as Stanford type B. Acute pain is the most common symptom, which can result from the dissection alone or the consequences of the dissection such as chest pain (involvement of coronary arteries), abdominal pain (involvement of coeliac or mesenteric arteries), back pain (involvement of renal arteries), or limb pain (involvement of the subclavian artery or common iliac arteries). Other symptoms include syncope, while examination may reveal signs of aortic regurgitation and cardiac tamponade. Neurological sequelae include stroke, Horner's syndrome, or acute paraplegia.

Musculoskeletal causes of acute severe back pain including acute disc prolapse or vertebral collapse may result in spinal cord compression or cauda equina syndrome, which are medical emergencies. Concerning symptoms suggestive of these conditions ('red flags') include bilateral sciatica, progressive neurological deficit, hesitancy in micturition, faecal and urinary incontinence, loss of anal tone, saddle anaesthesia, sudden spinal pain relieved by lying down, point tenderness over a vertebral body, or a structural deformity of the spine.

Intra-abdominal pathology such as pancreatitis, pyelonephritis, renal colic, and diverticulitis can be associated with back pain so careful abdominal examination is important, as well as consideration of blood tests e.g. amylase, and imaging. Splenic artery aneurysm rupture is a rare cause of upper abdominal pain which can be difficult to diagnose as early bleeding may be contained within the lesser sac meaning vital signs and haemoglobin may initially be normal.

Acute hypertension must prompt all clinicians to consider *hypertensive disorders of pregnancy* i.e. pre-eclampsia. This can be associated with important and potentially life-threatening complications such as hepatic subcapsular haemorrhage and capsular rupture which can cause severe pain.

Uterine rupture can cause upper abdominal pain due to intra-abdominal bleeding but would invariably be associated with fetal compromise and acute maternal collapse.

2. Why is this diagnosis more common in pregnancy?

Pregnancy increases the risk of arterial dissection because the vascular system is a lot more compliant during pregnancy. Microscopically, changes have been reported in the aortic media (including changes in the formation of elastic fibres, as well as smooth muscle hypertrophy and hyperplasia), and macroscopically there is a small increase in aortic diameter. Aortic dissection typically occurs in the third trimester or in the postpartum period when these changes are maximal.

3. What investigations would you arrange?

If a patient is stable enough to be transferred for imaging, then urgent cross-sectional imaging is crucial. The quickest way to confirm a suspicion of aortic dissection is with CT angiogram, but MR angiogram can also be used. If a patient is unstable, then echocardiography is an option, but this will not provide images of the entire aorta.

Whilst it is desirable to avoid ionizing radiation in pregnancy and use modalities such as ultrasound or MRI, there are some situations where this cannot be performed in the time required, or where CT is preferred to confirm or refute a potentially life-threatening diagnosis. CT can and should be performed in an emergency in pregnancy. The fetal dose from CT imaging of head and chest is under 1mGy, whereas the threshold for fetal consequences of radiation exposure is thought to be approximately 200 mGy. If lower abdominal imaging is required, then the risks to the fetus and the benefits to the mother should be evaluated, considering the urgency of the clinical situation and availability of alternatives; pregnancy is not an absolute contra-indication to abdominal CT. The mother can be reassured that intravenous contrast used for CT is safe in both pregnancy and breastfeeding.

In non-pregnant individuals with aortic dissection, a rise in D-dimer can be a sensitive marker of aortic dissection, however the normal rise in D-dimer levels seen in pregnancy mean that this is not advocated as part of any diagnostic assessment.

4. How would you manage this condition?

Acute dissection remains a rare but catastrophic complication and urgent delivery of the fetus and treatment of the dissection are essential in this patient, given her gestation. This patient requires optimization of antihypertensive treatment initially with oral or intravenous beta-blockade, and then planning of urgent surgical intervention. The woman should be managed where cardiothoracic and obstetric services are co-located. Urgent caesarean delivery is then performed with subsequent surgical treatment of the dissection.

5. What underlying genetic diagnoses must be considered?

Spontaneous aortic dissection in pregnancy has been reported, but meticulous clinical assessment for features of an underlying genetic diagnosis is crucial, as is genetic testing. Whilst the ideal situation is that any woman with a phenotype suggestive of the conditions below has a diagnosis made prior to conception (and therefore then has the opportunity for pre-pregnancy counselling), the reality is that often this diagnosis is not made until a significant complication occurs.

Marfan syndrome is an autosomal dominant disorder of connective tissue, secondary to a mutation in the fibrillin 1 (*FBN1*) gene, which subsequently affects both elastic and non-elastic fibres. It is diagnosed using the revised Ghent nosology, by the presence of an increased aortic diameter (based on a Z score), in combination with ectopia lentis or positive family history of a *FBN1* mutation, as well as systemic manifestations (including pectus carinatum, pneumothorax, mitral valve prolapse, scoliosis, and myopia).

Loeys–Dietz syndrome is a recently described genetic condition affecting connective tissue resulting from mutations in genes involved in the transforming growth factor beta pathway, which is important in growth and development and the formation of the extracellular matrix. It is an autosomal dominant condition, but a large proportion of individuals have *de novo* mutations, with no family history. It can lead to aortic dilatation, aneurysm and dissection, as well as dural ectasia, scoliosis, pneumothorax, and similar skin and joint manifestations to both Ehlers–Danlos syndrome and Marfan syndrome. The cardiac and vascular manifestations are the main cause for concern as they can occur at a younger age than those seen in Marfan syndrome (where aortic dissection is rarely seen in childhood).

Familial thoracic aortic aneurysm syndrome is a genetic condition characterized by mutations involved in connective tissue synthesis, associated with increased risk of dissection in pregnancy.

Ehlers–Danlos syndrome (EDS) is a group of genetic connective tissue disorders with signs and symptoms resulting from mutations in genes involved in the synthesis of collagen. They are characterized by joint hypermobility, skin and tissue fragility (with poor wound healing), and joint dislocations. The main concerning type for cardiovascular complications is type 4 ('vascular') EDS where aortic dissection, arterial rupture, spontaneous rupture of internal organs (bowel, uterus), and cardiac valve abnormalities have been described.

Further reading

1. **Zhu J** *et al.* Aortic dissection in pregnancy: Management strategy and outcomes. The Annals of Thoracic Surgery. 2017; **103**: 1199–206.
2. ESC guidelines for management of cardiac problems in pregnancy (2018). <https://www.escardio.org/Guidelines/Clinical-Practice-Guidelines/Cardiovascular-Diseases-during-Pregnancy-Management-of>

Case 2

A 26-year-old woman presented to the Emergency Department with a 10-day history of vomiting. Over the preceding 24 hours she had vomited approximately 10 times. She reported being unable to sustain any oral intake but had not had diarrhoea or abdominal pain. She had lost 5 kg of weight in the last few weeks (from a baseline of 52 kg). She has been diagnosed with asthma previously for which she used a regular steroid inhaler and a salbutamol inhaler when required. She was on no other regular medications.

A urinary pregnancy test was positive, and she thought her last menstrual period was 10 weeks previously.

Initial assessment

General inspection: Dehydrated
Heart rate: 105 bpm
Blood pressure: 90/65 mmHg
Respiratory rate: 16 breaths/min
Temperature: 36.4 °C
Oxygen saturations: 99% on room air
Urinalysis: 3+ ketones; No protein, nitrites, or blood

Examination

Cardiovascular: Normal heart sounds, no murmurs
Respiratory: Normal breath sounds
Abdomen: Soft, non-tender abdomen

Bloods

See Table 2.1.

Table 2.1 Bloods

Haemoglobin	124 g/L
WCC	5.23 × 10⁹/L
Platelets	376 × 10⁹/L
Sodium	139 mmol/L
Potassium	3.6 mmol/L
Urea	3.5 mmol/L
Creatinine	45 µmol/L
Bilirubin	6 µmol/L
ALT	36 iU/L
Albumin	38 g/L
Calcium	2.44 mmol/L
TSH	< 0.01 mu/L
fT4	25.2 pmol/L
fT3	6.9 pmol/L
CRP	16 mg/L
Amylase	104 U/L

Questions

1. What are the potential causes of her symptoms?
2. What is the cause of her abnormal thyroid function?
3. What additional tests should you request?
4. How could you treat her vomiting?
5. How do you treat her underlying condition?

Answers

1. What are the potential causes of her symptoms?

Vomiting can be caused by a wide variety of pathologies and a careful history and examination is required to clarify the likely cause. The duration of symptoms and her calculated gestational age make hyperemesis gravidarum the most likely diagnosis, but it is important to consider other causes of vomiting such as biliary disease, pancreatitis, and bowel obstruction.

2. What is the cause of her abnormal thyroid function?

Gestational thyrotoxicosis is seen in 1–3% of all pregnancies and is typically associated with hyperemesis gravidarum and multiple pregnancy. HCG is structurally similar to TSH and binds to TSH receptors on the thyroid gland, causing an increase in release of T3 and T4. These in turn suppress TSH production from the pituitary gland leading to a lower TSH. Women with gestational thyrotoxicosis do not have other symptoms of thyrotoxicosis. Gestational trophoblastic disease can cause particularly severe gestational thyrotoxicosis due to the high levels of HCG that can occur.

Graves' disease is autoimmune thyrotoxicosis, driven by TSH receptor antibodies which stimulate the thyroid. New diagnoses of Graves' disease are uncommon in pregnancy. Graves' disease is specifically associated with thyroid eye disease.

Toxic nodule/multinodular goitre can both be associated with hyperthyroidism but antibody testing is negative.

3. What additional tests should you request?

A careful history looking at a personal and family history of thyroid disease, thyroid eye disease, or autoimmune disease, in addition to clinical examination, can usually distinguish gestational from pathological hyperthyroidism. If there is a concern about underlying primary hyperthyroidism, TSH receptor antibodies can be measured, and if positive, confirm Grave's disease. There is no role for measuring TPO antibodies in hyperthyroidism. An ultrasound can help in the identification of a thyroid nodule or multinodular goitre but cannot confirm if these are hormonally active. Thyroid uptake scans should be avoided in pregnancy.

In all women with severe hyperemesis gravidarum, routine tests should include urinalysis, urine culture, FBC, renal function, electrolytes including calcium level, blood glucose level, thyroid function, liver function tests and amylase. A venous blood gas should be considered. An ultrasound is required to confirm the presence of a viable pregnancy and approximate gestational age, and this will importantly also identify a multiple pregnancy or molar pregnancy.

4. How could you treat her vomiting?

Medications are shown in Table 2.2.

Table 2.2 Medications

First line	H1 receptor antagonist: cyclizine OR promethazine Then add in phenothiazine: prochlorperazine OR chlorpromazine
Second line	D2 antagonist: metoclopramide OR domperidone (instead of, not in addition to, phenothiazines due to increased risk of side effects in combination) Then add in 5-HT3 receptor antagonist: ondansetron*
Third line	Steroids after discussion with senior obstetrician/obstetric physician

*Recent data suggest a small increase in risk of cleft lip/palate with use in the first trimester, so discussion of the potential risks and benefits to the individual is advised. <http://www.uktis.org/docs/Ondansetron%202019.pdf>

Reprinted from Collins S and Frise C. *Obstetric Medicine* (Oxford University Press, 2020) with permission from Oxford University Press.

If dehydrated, use 0.9% sodium chloride, with additional potassium if required, for rehydration. B vitamins, particularly thiamine, should also be given to women admitted to hospital with a prolonged duration of vomiting. If admitted for treatment, the woman should also be offered venous thromboembolism prophylaxis with LMWH (unless contra-indications are present).

The first-line antiemetics include H1 receptor antagonists and phenothiazines such as cyclizine, prochlorperazine, promethazine, and chlorpromazine. Metoclopramide and domperidone are second-line therapy as these have a risk of extrapyramidal effects and oculogyric crises. A combination tablet containing doxylamine (an antihistamine) and pyridoxine is the only licensed antiemetic for use in pregnancy and can be used in combination with other medications.

Ondansetron is a very effective antiemetic. One study showed an association with cleft palate in those women who used ondansetron in the first trimester (an additional 3 cases/10,000 pregnancies). Subsequent data have not supported this finding, so this information does not preclude its use in the first trimester; however appropriate counselling is advised.

It is usually more effective to add in a combination of antiemetics than to change between antiemetics. Corticosteroids can be considered where standard antiemetics have failed. A suggested regimen is intravenous hydrocortisone 100 mg twice daily, and if effective, converting to oral prednisolone 40–50 mg daily once tolerated. This should be tapered as symptoms resolve.

In addition, ginger and acupressure have both been found to help nausea and vomiting in pregnancy.

5. How do you manage her underlying condition?

Gestational thyrotoxicosis can be managed in a supportive fashion until thyroid function improves. Hydration and antiemetics will help with nausea and vomiting.

Antithyroid drugs would be advised if it became clear that the thyroid dysfunction was resulting from Grave's disease, e.g. if signs of hyperthyroidism are present, TSH receptor antibodies are positive, or the thyroid function worsens with increasing gestation even when hyperemesis improves.

Both propylthiouracil (PTU) and carbimazole are associated with an increase in risk of congenital malformations. Approximately 10 additional cases of congenital malformations per 1000 births to women exposed to PTU in pregnancy are encountered, compared to an additional 17 cases of congenital malformations per 1000 births in pregnancies exposed to carbimazole/methimazole, and a higher rate still if both agents are used in pregnancy. It should be noted that untreated hyperthyroidism also results in approximately 10 additional cases of congenital abnormalities per 1000 births. PTU is associated with up to a 6% risk of severe maternal liver disease, whereas the risk of maternal side effects with carbimazole is lower. Women on either type of antithyroid medication should be advised about the risk of agranulocytosis and therefore to monitor carefully for infection. A full blood count is required urgently if any symptoms of infection develop whilst taking this medication.

Further reading

1. **T. Korevaar** *et al.* Thyroid disease in pregnancy: New insights in clinical diagnosis and management. Nature Reviews Endocrinology. 2017; **13**: 610–22.
2. **M. Agrawal** *et al.* Antithyroid drug therapy in pregnancy and risk of congenital anomalies: Systematic review and meta-analysis. Clinical Endocrinology. 2022; 96: 857–868.

Case 3

A 28-year-old woman with no known medical problems presented with a 9-day history of a non-productive cough, shortness of breath, fever, headache, and loss of smell and taste. She was 35 weeks into her first pregnancy. She had not been abroad recently. She lived with her husband and his parents, and all had developed similar symptoms in the preceding few days. Her booking BP was 110/80 mmHg and BMI was 30 kg/m². She was not on any regular medication, there was no family history of medical problems, and she had never smoked. She was of Indian ethnicity and had decided not to be vaccinated against SARS-CoV2 whilst she was pregnant.

Initial assessment

General inspection: Unwell, breathless
Heart rate: 120 bpm
Blood pressure: 98/55 mmHg
Respiratory rate: 30 breaths/min
Temperature: 38.7 °C
Oxygen saturations: 88% on room air
Urinalysis: No protein, 2+ ketones

Examination

Cardiovascular: Normal heart sounds, no murmurs
Respiratory: Bilateral crackles
Abdomen: Soft abdomen, non-tender gravid uterus

Bloods

See Table 3.1.

Arterial blood gas (on air)

See Table 3.2.

Investigations

CXR   Diffuse interstitial shadowing bilaterally.
ECG   Sinus tachycardia.

Table 3.1 Bloods

Haemoglobin	110 g/L
WCC	6.5×10^9/L
Neutrophils	5.7×10^9/L
Lymphocytes	0.6×10^9/L
Platelets	300×10^9/L
Sodium	134 mmol/L
Potassium	3.5 mmol/L
Urea	7 mmol/L
Creatinine	50 µmol/L
Bilirubin	6 µmol/L
ALT	100 iU/L
ALP	110 iU/L
Albumin	29 g/L
CRP	300 mg/L

Table 3.2 Arterial blood gas

pH	7.36
PaO_2	7.5 kPa
$PaCO_2$	5.6 kPa
HCO_3^-	22 mmol/L
Base excess	−3 mmol/L

Questions

1. What are the potential causes of her signs and symptoms?
2. What further investigations would you like to do?
3. What would your initial management of this patient be?

Answers

1. What are the potential causes of her signs and symptoms?

The history, examination, and investigations are consistent with a severe respiratory tract infection, and several causative organisms should be considered.

Viral infection

COVID-19 (infection with SARS-CoV2) is most likely given her symptoms, and in addition to pregnancy alone, she has several features that put her more at risk of severe infection, including her ethnicity and BMI. Her symptoms overlap with those of other non-COVID viral infections, but prominent headache and a loss of sense of smell and/or taste are more specific for COVID-19. Symptoms, however, depend on the exact variant of the virus, so should be interpreted with knowledge about the commonest variants locally in mind. She has not been vaccinated, which increases the risk of severe infection requiring hospitalization and intensive care admission.

Influenza should always be considered in women with these symptoms, and as with COVID-19, infection in pregnancy is associated with a higher mortality compared to the non-pregnant population, and underlying medical problems increase the chance of more severe infection.

Varicella zoster primary infection in pregnancy is associated with a higher incidence of pneumonitis, and a careful inspection looking for a vesicular rash should be undertaken in addition to assessment of any potential recent exposure.

Other respiratory viruses such as adenovirus and respiratory syncytial virus should be considered, as well as MERS (Middle Eastern Respiratory Syndrome) and SARS (Severe Acute Respiratory Syndrome) which should be considered if there is suggestive travel history, depending on prevalence data.

Bacterial infection

Bacterial and viral chest infections are difficult to distinguish clinically. Focal consolidation is more common in bacterial infection than bilateral diffuse infiltrates. Procalcitonin can help in distinguishing viral and bacterial infection. Common causative organisms are the same as those in the non-pregnant population, and include *Streptococcus pneumonia*, *Staphylococcus aureus*, *Klebsiella pneumoniae*, and *Haemophilus influenzae* as well as atypical organisms such as *Mycoplasma pneumonia* and *Legionella pneumonia*. In addition, organisms such as *Listeria monocytogenes* should be considered, as although rare as a cause for respiratory symptoms, infection in pregnancy has fetal implications including chorioamnionitis, preterm labour, miscarriage, or stillbirth.

Pulmonary tuberculosis usually presents with chronic respiratory symptoms such as cough and haemoptysis, as well as with systemic features such as night sweats, weight loss, and lymphadenopathy. Untreated, this can be associated with fetal growth restriction.

Fungal infection

Pneumocystis jirovecii is a rare cause of pneumonia, where hypoxia can be significant, that should be considered in individuals on long-term immunosuppressive agents, with malignancy (haematological or non-haematological) or HIV, or those receiving chemotherapy.

2. What further investigations would you like to do?

Tests for the causative organism include viral swabs (SARS-CoV2, respiratory virus screen), blood cultures, early morning sputum samples if TB is being considered, and urine for pneumococcal and/or legionella antigens. Even with rigorous testing the causative organism may not be identified. It would also be important to ascertain her HIV status if not already known.

Cross-sectional imaging with CT can also be considered. This is not required in all those with a viral or bacterial respiratory infection but can be useful if there is additional concern about co-existent pulmonary emboli (particularly given the thrombotic risk of COVID-19 infection) or complications of the infection such as abscess formation, pleural infection, or pneumothorax.

3. What would your initial management of this patient be?

Concern about COVID-19 infection means that all healthcare professionals involved in her care should be wearing personal protective equipment in line with local guidelines.

Management of women with confirmed COVID-19 should follow local and national guidelines. Priorities include:

(1) Oxygen supplementation as needed to maintain oxygen saturations at the target (guidelines usually have a higher target for pregnant women compared to non-pregnant individuals) with escalation to nasal cannulae, face mask, non-invasive ventilatory support (mainly continuous positive airway pressure), invasive ventilation, and extra-corporeal membrane oxygenation as required.

(2) Corticosteroids in women requiring oxygen. Oral prednisolone or IV hydrocortisone is preferred for maternal indications like this as far less is transported across the placenta compared to dexamethasone.

(3) Additional treatments for COVID-19 (such as tocilizumab, REGEN-COV monoclonal antibodies, sotrovimab) as per national guidance.

(4) Antibiotics if there is a concern about bacterial infection.

(5) VTE prophylaxis with LMWH if no contraindications are present, increased to intermediate or treatment dose LMWH in accordance with local or national guidance and cross-sectional imaging if deemed clinically appropriate.

Women should be reviewed daily by a multidisciplinary team with experience in managing acutely unwell pregnant women (such as a senior obstetrician, physician, obstetric physician, anaesthetist, and intensivist) to decide on appropriate methods of fetal monitoring, whether delivery needs to be expedited (and if so whether steroids for fetal lung maturation are required) as well as practical considerations such as where the woman should be cared for.

Further reading

1. RCOG Coronavirus (COVID-19) infection and pregnancy guidance
   <https://www.rcog.org.uk/coronavirus-pregnancy>

Case 4

A 33-year-old woman in her second pregnancy presented to the maternity assessment unit at 37 weeks of gestation with a 3-day history of itching and a new rash. She initially noticed the rash on the right side of her abdomen. It then spread across her abdomen, to involve both arms and legs, and neck. The rash was very itchy. She had had a cough and coryzal symptoms a week previously, but symptoms had resolved, and she had no temperature or other symptoms at that time. Oral antihistamines had not relieved the itching. She had a history of eczema, but this normally only affected her hands. She has tried her normal emollient, but this did not help.

Initial assessment

General inspection:	Well, but uncomfortable
Heart rate;	70 bpm
Blood pressure:	105/78 mmHg
Respiratory rate:	16 breaths/min
Temperature:	36.7 °C
Oxygen saturations:	98% on room air
Urinalysis:	No protein

Examination

Cardiovascular:	Normal heart sounds, no murmurs
Respiratory:	Normal breath sounds
Abdomen:	Soft abdomen, non-tender gravid uterus
Skin:	Widespread papular erythematous rash over the abdomen (sparing umbilicus), chest, neck, upper arms, and thighs
	Excoriation marks at the edges and some rough plaque formation over the abdomen; no vesicles or bullae

Bloods

See Table 4.1.

Table 4.1 Bloods

Haemoglobin	128 g/L
WCC	4.3 × 10⁹/L
Platelets	175 × 10⁹/L
Sodium	136 mmol/L
Potassium	3.8 mmol/L
Urea	2.2 mmol/L
Creatinine	40 μmol/L
Bilirubin	6 μmol/L
ALT	25 iU/L
ALP	100 iU/L
Albumin	29 g/L
CRP	12 mg/L

Questions

1. What potential diagnoses are you considering?
2. What investigations would you arrange?
3. What treatment would you offer?
4. How would you counsel the patient about the use of oral steroids in pregnancy?

Answers

1. What potential diagnoses are you considering?

Polymorphic eruption of pregnancy (PEP), formerly known as PUPPP (pruritic urticarial papules and plaques of pregnancy), presents with pruritic, erythematous papules. The itch may precede the rash. Small fluid-filled blisters can form, which leak clear fluid. The rash may coalesce and form plaques or target lesions. The rash typically starts on the abdomen within striae, and characteristically spares the umbilicus. It can spread across the trunk, abdomen, under the breasts, and on to the limbs. The palms, soles, face, and scalp are rarely affected.

PEP usually occurs in the late third trimester or in the early postpartum. It affects 1 in 160–300 pregnancies. It is more common in nulliparous women and in multiple pregnancies, seemingly due to overdistension of the skin. It typically resolves in 4–6 weeks and rarely recurs in future pregnancies.

PEP has no effect on the fetus and should not impact on the timing or method of childbirth.

Pemphigoid gestationis (PG) is a rare pregnancy-specific dermatosis, affecting between 1 in 1700–50,000 pregnancies. It is an autoimmune condition, associated with haplotypes HLA-DR3 and HLA-DR4, and diagnosis is confirmed by skin biopsy. It usually occurs in the third trimester and rarely after childbirth. The rash appears on the abdomen, often around the umbilicus. It starts as papules and plaques with large, tense bullae forming within a few weeks. The rash extends across the abdomen, trunk, and limbs. The palms and soles may be involved but the mucosal membranes are spared. It may improve towards the end of pregnancy but as with other autoimmune conditions, often flares after birth. It may recur in subsequent pregnancies.

PG has implications for the fetus. Intrauterine growth restriction has been reported in women with PG so serial growth scans for fetal assessment should be discussed and offered to the woman. In addition the antibodies can cross the placenta so approximately 10% of infants develop a mild, self-limiting rash.

Atopic eruption of pregnancy, also known as prurigo gestationis or eczema of pregnancy, is a benign condition affecting 1 in 300 women. It presents as erythematous excoriated nodules or papules on the face, neck, chest, trunk, and extensor surfaces of the limbs. This is more common in women with a personal of family history of atopy and can occur at any point in pregnancy, but is most often seen in women in the second trimester. It has no effect on the fetus.

Pustular psoriasis of pregnancy is a very rare variant of generalized pustular psoriasis. It can occur at any time but typically in the third trimester or early postpartum. It presents as erythematous plaques studded with sterile pustules. The rash typically starts in the intertriginous areas and spreads centrally, sparing the face, palms, and soles. Pustular psoriasis of pregnancy does not usually cause pruritus but is often associated with systemic symptoms such as fatigue, fever, diarrhoea, and delirium. It is associated with intrauterine growth restriction, miscarriage, and stillbirth so the fetus should be closely monitored.

Allergic reactions are also a rarer cause of a presentation like this.

2. What investigations would you perform?

The dermatoses of pregnancy are typically diagnosed on clinical history and exam-ination, however the following tests are suggested for all women with significant pruritus and a rash:

- FBC and CRP: inflammatory markers are elevated in pustular psoriasis of pregnancy.
- Bile acids and liver function tests: cholestatic conditions such as intrahepatic cholestasis of pregnancy can cause itching (but not a primary rash)
- Thyroid function: pemphigoid gestationis is associated with other autoimmune conditions so should check for autoimmune thyroid disease.
- Skin biopsy is occasionally required

3. What treatment would you offer?

For polymorphic eruption of pregnancy, treatment options include:

- Topical emollients and soap substitutes hydrate and provide a barrier for the inflamed skin.
- 1% menthol in aqueous cream, calamine lotion, cool baths, and ice packs are all options that may soothe the symptoms of itching.
- Mid- or high-potency topical steroids (e.g. betamethasone 0.05%).
- Antihistamines can help improve pruritus.
- Oral prednisolone may be required in severe cases, and usually results in an im-provement in symptoms in a few days.

4. How would you counsel her about the use of oral steroids in pregnancy?

The woman should be reassured that oral prednisolone is safe and appropriate to use in pregnancy. Prednisolone is metabolized to inactive cortisone by 11 beta-hydroxysteroid dehydrogenase in the placenta. Therefore only 10% or less of the active drug reaches the fetus. This contrasts with other steroids such as dexa-methasone and betamethasone, which are not metabolized by the placenta and therefore cross to the fetus to a much greater degree. In contrast to prednisolone which is preferred for the treatment of maternal conditions, dexamethasone and betamethasone are therefore used in preference for treatment of fetal conditions and to aid fetal lung maturation if preterm birth is anticipated.

There were studies in the 1950s and 1990s that reported an increased risk of cleft palate with oral corticosteroid use. However, subsequent larger and better controlled studies have found no association between antenatal corticosteroid use and congenital anomalies. Any other reports of adverse effects from antenatal corticosteroids, such as intrauterine growth restriction or preterm birth, are confounded by the existence of the maternal disease that the steroids were being used to treat. Therefore, women should be advised that untreated inflammatory conditions are of greater risk in pregnancy than using steroids to treat them.

Further reading

1. C. Savervall *et al.* Dermatological diseases associated with pregnancy: Pemphigoid gestationis, polymorphic eruption of pregnancy, intrahepatic cholestasis of pregnancy, and atopic eruption of pregnancy. Dermatology Research and Practice. 2015; **2015**: 979635. doi:10.1155/2015/979635.

Case 5

A 36-year-old woman presented in spontaneous labour at 40 weeks of gestation. This was her first pregnancy and it had been uneventful up to this point. She had no past medical history and was on no regular medications except multivitamins. She worked as a lawyer, did not smoke, drink alcohol, or take recreational drugs. She was a keen cyclist and had exercised throughout pregnancy.

On admission her blood pressure was 108/64 mmHg and her urine showed 2+ ketones. During the following 12 hours she was given 2L of intravenous 5% glucose. She appeared to be a bit vague during labour, and was not always following the instructions of her midwife. Her husband was present and encouraged her throughout, including ensuring she drank 1L of water every 3 hours.

She delivered a female infant vaginally. Apgar scores were 5, 6, and 10 at 1, 5, and 10 minutes respectively. Shortly after birth the baby had a tonic-clonic seizure, requiring intubation and ventilation and was transferred to the neonatal intensive care unit. The umbilical cord blood gas samples showed a sodium of 114 mmol/L.

Initial assessment

General inspection: Well hydrated, confused, agitated
Heart rate: 60 bpm
Blood pressure: 115/70 mmHg
Respiratory rate: 18 breaths/min
Temperature: 37.1 °C
Oxygen saturations: 98% on room air
Urinalysis: No protein, no ketones

Examination

Cardiovascular: Normal heart sounds, no murmurs
Respiratory: Normal breath sounds
Abdomen: Soft abdomen, well-contracted uterus
Neurology: GCS 14 (E4, M6, V4)
Normal cranial nerves
All limbs: normal tone, power, reflexes, sensation
Unable to assess coordination due to difficulty following instructions

Venous blood gas

See Table 5.1.

Table 5.1 Venous blood gas

pH	7.33
Sodium	118 mmol/L
Potassium	3.7 mmol/L
Base excess	−3.3 mmol/L
Chloride	100 mmol/L
Lactate	2.2 mmol/L
Glucose	4.2 mmol/L

Questions

1. What causes of acute confusion do you need to consider?
2. What contributes to hyponatraemia in the intrapartum period?
3. What investigations would you undertake?
4. How would you manage this condition?

Answers

1. What causes of acute confusion do you need to consider?

Acute hyponatremia is seen here, with a very low maternal and neonatal sodium, sufficient to explain both the maternal symptoms and neonatal seizure. This may have severe neurological consequences including seizures, encephalopathy, and cognitive dysfunction.

Cerebral venous sinus thrombosis is more common in pregnancy compared to the general population due to the increase in prothrombotic coagulation factors. Headache is the most common symptom, however it can also present as encephalopathy with disturbances of consciousness and cognitive dysfunction. Seizures (focal or generalized), intracranial hypertension, and focal neurology such as oculomotor palsies can also occur.

An unwitnessed seizure can result in confusion after the seizure has terminated, in the 'post-ictal' phase, where drowsiness is also common. A seizure can result from many different pathologies in pregnancy, including acute hyponatraemia. Occurrence of a seizure should always be considered, but as there was no witnessed history of this from the people with her throughout, this seems unlikely in this case.

Posterior reversible encephalopathy syndrome (PRES) is a neurological syndrome defined by specific clinical and radiological features (characteristic changes on MRI), the cause of which is uncertain but is likely to be due to dysfunctional cerebral autoregulation and endothelial dysfunction. In pregnancy this usually co-exists with hypertension. Neurological symptoms include headache, altered consciousness (which can vary from confusion and agitation to coma), visual disturbance including cortical blindness and seizures.

Intrapartum sepsis is common, and any infection may cause confusion. Sources of sepsis may be pregnancy-specific such as chorioamnionitis, or unrelated to the pregnancy, for example pneumonia or meningitis.

2. What contributes to hyponatremia in the intrapartum period?

In healthy pregnancy there is activation of the renin-aldosterone system, as well as increased oxytocin release which has similar structure to vasopressin and therefore has an anti-diuretic effect. There is also a change in the sensitivity of the hypothalamic osmoreceptors. Overall this causes physiological volume expansion, leading to a fall in serum sodium and average plasma osmolality between the first trimester and the third. These changes in the normal range must be remembered when reviewing a pregnant woman with hyponatraemia.

There are numerous causes of hyponatraemia in non-pregnant individuals. In addition, dilutional hyponatraemia and pre-eclampsia are the main causes of hyponatraemia in pregnancy.

Dilutional hyponatraemia is the most likely cause for hyponatraemia in this case. Excessive fluid intake, either oral or intravenous, is a risk factor for hyponatraemia, with women receiving more than 2.5 L of fluid in labour being 16 times more likely to develop hyponatraemia than those receiving less than 1L of fluid. Oxytocin use and prolonged labour are also associated with hyponatraemia.

Pre-eclampsia can also be associated with hyponatraemia, with low sodium seen in approximately one-third of cases. The underlying pathophysiology is not fully understood but may be due to extravascular fluid shifts as a result of altered capillary permeability, and/or inappropriate ADH release and subsequent excessive water retention.

3. What investigations would you undertake?

Clinical assessment of fluid status is key in diagnosing the cause of hyponatraemia. Pregnant women should have the same clinical assessment as non-pregnant women, including capillary refill, heart rate, blood pressure, jugular venous pressure, mucous membranes, and skin turgor.

With all cases of hyponatraemia, investigations to consider include:

- Paired serum and urine sodium and osmolality
- Renal function
- Thyroid function
- 9am cortisol
- Liver function including albumin
- Blood glucose

A low threshold for cranial imaging with either CT or MRI is advised, depending on the exact clinical history and chronology of events.

4. How would you manage this condition?

Most cases of dilutional hyponatraemia can be managed by avoiding any extra fluids and encouraging the woman to drink only if thirsty. She will rapidly clear the extra free water. As the hyponatraemia is acute (within 12 hours), there is a very low risk of central pontine myelinolysis during correction of hyponatraemia.

In severe dilutional hyponatraemia where the woman has significant neurological symptoms (e.g. reduced GCS, is obtunded, or having seizures) then a bolus of hypertonic sodium chloride can be given and repeated until either symptoms improve or the sodium increases by a maximum of 10 mmol/l. This is rarely required in practice, however.

To prevent hyponatraemia in labour, it is advisable to avoid excessive oral and unnecessary intravenous fluids, alongside encouragement of the women only to drink to thirst. Careful fluid balance recording is recommended, with consideration of bloods for sodium measurement if the woman receives more than about 1500 ml of fluid in labour.

Further reading

1. Guideline for the prevention, diagnosis and management of hyponatraemia in labour and the immediate postpartum period, the regulation and quality improvement authority (March 2017). <https://www.rqia.org.uk/RQIA/files/df/dfd57ddd-ceb3-4c0d-9719-8e33e179d0ff.pdf>

2. S. Xodo *et al*. Preeclampsia and low sodium: A retrospective cohort analysis and literature review. Pregnancy Hypertension. 2021; 23, 1690173.

Case 6

A 45-year-old woman with no past medical history presented with a painful left thigh, 4 weeks after the birth of her first child. The pain started 3 days prior to presentation on the medial aspect of the thigh, and subsequently radiated down the leg. It was associated with erythema, mild swelling, and pain on palpation. There was no history of trauma, no associated pain elsewhere, and she had never experienced anything similar in the past. Her pregnancy had been uncomplicated, but she had required an emergency caesarean delivery for a failed induction of labour. She had received 10 days of LMWH as VTE prophylaxis and had taken all the doses as prescribed. She had tried paracetamol with limited effect. She was not on any regular medications and had no significant family history. She had never smoked.

Initial assessment

General inspection:	Looks well
Heart rate:	90 bpm
Blood pressure:	135/85 mmHg
Respiratory rate:	16 breaths/min
Temperature:	36.9 °C
Oxygen saturations:	99% on room air
Urinalysis:	Negative

Examination

Cardiovascular:	Normal heart sounds, no murmurs
Respiratory:	Normal breath sounds
Abdomen:	Soft, no tenderness, caesarean section wound healing well
Left leg:	Erythema on medial thigh, with a palpable more solid area of approximately 10 cm in length, along the course of the long saphenous vein
Right leg:	No swelling, tenderness, or erythema

Bloods

See Table 6.1.

Table 6.1 Bloods

Haemoglobin	125 g/L
WCC	12×10^9/L
Platelets	350×10^9/L
Sodium	135 mmol/L
Potassium	4.1 mmol/L
Urea	3.6 mmol/L
Creatinine	45 μmol/L
Bilirubin	12 μmol/L
ALT	20 iU/L
Albumin	28g/L
CRP	23 mg/L

Questions

1. Which potential causes of her symptoms should be considered?
2. What other investigations would you like to perform?
3. What treatment options exist?

Answers

1. Which potential causes of her symptoms should be considered?

Superficial phlebitis/superficial thrombophlebitis is the most likely cause of her symptoms. Superficial phlebitis is inflammation of a superficial vein that is not associated with thrombosis in that vein. If there is associated thrombosis in a tributary vein, then this constitutes superficial thrombophlebitis. A higher risk of deep venous thrombus is associated with superficial venous thrombus within 3 cm of the saphenofemoral junction, a thrombus of 5 cm or more in length, reduced mobility, a lack of association with varicose veins, or a history of DVT, PE, or active cancer.

Presentation is with a painful lump or erythema, which may follow the course of the vein. As with all thromboses, this is most common in the postpartum period. An ultrasound is required to confirm the diagnosis and assess the extent of the abnormal area, as well as whether co-existent deep venous thrombosis is present.

Deep vein thrombosis (DVT) is also an important differential to consider. DVT can present with symptoms of pain, swelling, and erythema, but does not often lead to a palpable lump in this area.

Haematoma can cause similar symptoms and can be spontaneous (e.g. related to an underlying bleeding tendency or anticoagulant medication), or secondary to trauma.

Cellulitis can cause a similar clinical picture. Symptoms may include fever, erythema, broken skin, or evidence of a bite, severe pain, and features of sepsis if severe, including hypotension and tachycardia. Necrotising fasciitis is a medical emergency and should be considered if pain is out of proportion to the evidence of localized infection. Group A streptococcus is of particular concern in pregnancy (see Case 37) so appropriate antibiotics should be given urgently.

2. What other investigations would you like to perform?

Venous Doppler ultrasound of the relevant leg is important for looking at both superficial and deep veins, and sometimes may be beneficial in identifying other localized pathology. It is important to remember that standard investigation for DVT only looks at veins of the upper leg, so if the symptoms are localized to a specific or different area, this should be clearly stated at the time of the request, so that if appropriate, the healthcare professional performing the ultrasound can assess that area also. *D-dimer* level is affected by pregnancy so this should not be used to aid decision-making about the likelihood of venous thromboembolism.

3. What treatment options exist?

Superficial thrombophlebitis is treated with analgesia, elevation of the affected limb, and consideration of compression stockings. Non-steroid anti-inflammatories can also be used before 28 weeks of gestation or postpartum. Patients should be encouraged to mobilize as normal. Anticoagulation with LMWH should be considered in those with higher risk lesions (as above) or with other risk factors for VTE.

Further reading

1. RCOG: Thrombosis and embolism during pregnancy and the puerperium, reducing the risk. (Green top Guideline 37a). (2015). <https://www.rcog.org.uk/en/guidelines-research-services/guidelines/gtg37a/>

2. NICE Clinical knowledge summary on superficial vein thrombosis. <https://cks.nice.org.uk/topics/superficial-vein-thrombosis-superficial-thrombophlebitis/management/management-of-superficial-vein-thrombosis/>

Case 7

A 22-year-old woman in her first pregnancy presented at 24 weeks of gestation with acute shortness of breath, which had developed over the preceding 24 hours. She described chest tightness, but no associated palpitations, cough, fever, or coryzal symptoms. She had had no previous similar episodes. Past medical history was notable for allergic rhinitis and childhood eczema and asthma. She was taking antacids when required for heartburn and was not on any regular medication. She had no family history of significant illnesses and had never smoked.

Initial assessment

General inspection:	Unwell, short of breath, wheezy
Heart rate:	115 bpm
Blood pressure:	117/70 mmHg
Respiratory rate:	30 breaths/min
Temperature:	36.8 °C
Oxygen saturations:	95% on room air
Urinalysis:	No protein

Examination

Cardiovascular:	Normal heart sounds, no murmurs
Respiratory:	Widespread wheeze, breath sounds bilaterally
	Peak expiratory flow rate 250 L/min
Abdomen:	Soft abdomen, non-tender gravid uterus

Bloods

See Table 7.1.

Table 7.1 Bloods

Haemoglobin	125 g/L
WCC	14.2 × 10⁹/L
Platelets	255 × 10⁹/L
Sodium	138 mmol/L
Potassium	3.8 mmol/L
Urea	2.8 mmol/L
Creatinine	50 μmol/L
Bilirubin	6 μmol/L
ALT	7 iU/L
ALP	70 iU/L
Albumin	34 g/L
CRP	20 mg/L

Questions

1. What are the potential causes of her symptoms?
2. What other investigations would you like to perform?
3. What investigation would help you confirm the diagnosis?
4. How would you treat this woman in the acute setting?
5. Which maintenance treatments might she benefit from in pregnancy?

Answers

1. What are the potential causes of her symptoms?

Asthma is a common cause of breathlessness and wheeze in women of childbearing age. Wheeze, breathlessness, and reduced peak flow rate (compared to predicted value for height, age, and sex) are characteristic of asthma, and a history of atopy is often associated. A new diagnosis of asthma in pregnancy is unusual and other diagnoses should be carefully looked for. A history of potential triggers should also be explored, for example occupational exposure to allergens, or hayfever symptoms.

Pulmonary oedema can cause wheezing, and is commonly misdiagnosed as asthma in pregnancy for this reason, particularly in women with no obvious predisposing risk factors for cardiac disease. Cardiogenic causes of pulmonary oedema in pregnancy include peripartum cardiomyopathy, valvular disease, and undiagnosed congenital heart disease. Pulmonary oedema is also seen in pre-eclampsia, after use of tocolytic medications, or following administration of excessive intravenous fluids.

Anaphylaxis is important to consider in someone presenting with acute wheeze and haemodynamic compromise. There may be an obvious trigger, particularly in those with a known allergy; however, anaphylaxis can still occur in the absence of an obvious trigger or allergy history. A thorough history, including drug history, is vital.

Other causes such as bronchiectasis, tracheal disease (although this more commonly causes stridor), and mediastinal masses may occasionally present with wheeze.

2. What other investigations would you like to perform?

Arterial blood gas (ABG) is essential in cases where there is concern about respiratory compromise. A high $PaCO_2$ is a sign of life-threatening asthma. Importantly the physiological changes in normal pregnancy mean the resting $PaCO_2$ in pregnancy is lower than in non-pregnant individuals, so a lower reference range should be used.

Chest radiography can help in the diagnosis of infection or pulmonary oedema.

Viral swabs for SARS-CoV-2, influenza, and other respiratory viruses should be considered.

Echocardiography is needed if there is any concern about an underlying cardiac cause of wheeze.

3. What investigation would help you confirm the diagnosis?

Spirometry is useful in the outpatient setting. In obstructive lung diseases such as asthma, the forced expiratory volume in 1 second (FEV1) is reduced and the forced vital capacity is normal or slightly reduced. This results in a FEV1/FVC ratio of less than 0.7. Other causes of an obstructive spirometry result include chronic obstructive pulmonary disease and bronchiectasis. Spirometry can be performed as normal in pregnancy.

The diagnosis of asthma requires a thorough history and the demonstration of reversibility of bronchoconstriction on spirometry. FeNO (fractional exhaled nitric oxide) testing is being increasingly performed in pregnant women to help guide management, as this is an indirect marker of airway inflammation. It is a simple, non-invasive test and can identify individuals who are more likely to respond to inhaled corticosteroids.

4. How would you treat this woman in the acute setting?

This woman has signs consistent with acute severe asthma (see Table 7.2 for classification). Treatment of acute asthma in pregnancy is the same as in non-pregnant individuals, and includes supplemental oxygen, nebulized bronchodilators (salbutamol, ipratropium bromide), oral or intravenous steroids, intravenous magnesium sulphate, and intravenous aminophylline.

Fetal monitoring should be performed given her gestation, and intervention for the benefit of the fetus should be delayed until the mother is stable.

Table 7.2 Assessing severity of acute asthma

Moderate acute asthma	• ↑ symptoms • PEF > 50–75% best or predicted • No features of acute severe asthma
Acute severe asthma	• Any one of: • PEF 33–50% best or predicted • Respiratory rate ≥ 25/min • Heart rate ≥ 110/min • Inability to complete sentences in 1 breath
Life-threatening asthma	**Any of the following in a ♀ with severe asthma**

	Clinical signs	Measurements
	• Altered conscious level	• PEF < 33% best or predicted
	• Exhaustion	• SpO_2 < 92%
	• Arrhythmia	• PaO_2 < 8 kPa
	• Hypotension	• 'Normal' $PaCO_2$ (4.6–6.0 kPa)*
	• Cyanosis	
	• Silent chest	
	• Poor respiratory effort	

Near-fatal asthma	Raised $PaCO_2$ and/or requiring mechanical intubation with raised inflation pressures

Reproduced from the British Thoracic Society and Scottish Intercollegiate Guidelines Network (2016) *SIGN 153: British guideline on the management of asthma: A national clinical guideline*: Edinburgh with kind permission.

* This is the non-pregnant reference range; we advise using lower reference range in pregnancy.

5. Which maintenance treatments might she benefit from in pregnancy?

Maintenance treatment of asthma in pregnancy follows the same stepwise approach as outside of pregnancy. Short- and long-acting beta-2 agonists, inhaled corticosteroids, leukotriene receptor antagonists, long-acting muscarinic receptor antagonists (tiotropium) and theophyllines are safe in pregnancy. Treatment for possible exacerbating factors should also be considered, such as treatment for hayfever, postnasal drip, or gastro-oesophageal reflux.

Further reading

1. **S. Karrasch** *et al*. Accuracy of FeNO testing for diagnosing asthma: a systematic review. Thorax. 2017; **72**: 109–16.

2. BTS/ SIGN British guideline on the management of asthma (2019). <https://www.brit-thoracic. org.uk/quality-improvement/guidelines/asthma/>

Case 8

A 45-year-old woman presented to the Emergency Department with a 3-day history of severe headache. She described some visual changes and nausea. Her past medical history was notable for infertility, for which she had undergone numerous investigations and three unsuccessful IVF cycles. She had a history of gastro-oesophageal reflux for which she took omeprazole daily. She had a family history of hypertension in both her parents and her older sister. She worked as an accountant. She had smoked 20 cigarettes a day for many years but stopped 1 year prior to this presentation. She drank 15–20 units of alcohol a week.

Initial assessment

General inspection: Body weight 130 kg
Heart rate: 90 bpm
Blood pressure: 200/130 mmHg
Temperature: 36.2 °C
Oxygen saturations: 99%
Urinalysis: 3+ protein, 2+ blood

Examination

Cardiovascular: Normal heart sounds
Respiratory: Normal breath sounds
Abdomen: Some mild epigastric tenderness
Fundoscopy: Some arteriolar narrowing bilaterally

Bloods

See Table 8.1.

She was admitted to hospital and an initial diagnosis of malignant hypertension and probable alcoholic liver disease was made. She was given oral ramipril. The night doctor is asked to review her as her blood pressure remained elevated. In response to his question about whether she could be pregnant, she describes amenorrhoea for several months which she attributed to being menopausal. A urinary pregnancy test is performed which is positive.

Table 8.1 Bloods

Haemoglobin	99 g/L
WCC	12 × 10⁹/L
Platelets	110 × 10⁹/L
Sodium	133 mmol/L
Potassium	3.6 mmol/L
Urea	2.1 mmol/L
Creatinine	100 μmol/L
Bilirubin	20 μmol/L
ALT	100 iU/L
ALP	200 iU/L
Albumin	31 g/L

Questions

1. How quickly would you refer her to obstetric care?
2. What other tests would you arrange?
3. Her blood pressure remains elevated despite the oral treatment, so what treatment would you give next?
4. Would you give her LMWH for VTE prophylaxis?

Answers

1. How quickly would you refer her to obstetric care?

She requires an immediate referral to the obstetric team given the constellation of symptoms, signs and laboratory abnormalities suggestive of a hypertensive disorder of pregnancy, and to confirm the presence of a pregnancy as well as gestational age. This will enable quick decisions to be made about appropriate fetal monitoring, maternal treatment including optimal control of her hypertension, location of care, and potential interventions that may be required.

2. What other tests would you arrange?

Pregnancy confirmation using an ultrasound is required urgently. Urinary HCG testing is very sensitive, so a serum HCG is not routinely required to confirm pregnancy. False negative results for both urinary and serum HCG can be seen in early pregnancy due to the 'hook effect' where very high levels of HCG molecules mean both the free and bound antibodies are saturated and no longer able to form the sandwich complexes read by the assay. HCG levels decline later in pregnancy, but this is uncommonly so low that it results in a negative urinary HCG result.

Blood tests including renal function, liver function, LDH, and a blood film are advised to assess for consequences of hypertension and features of pre-eclampsia/HELLP to enable a clear diagnosis to be made.

Urinalysis including microscopy is important, to look for red cells and casts which would be suggestive of underlying renal disease (a cause of the hypertension) or end-organ renal damage (a consequence of the hypertension).

Urine protein:creatinine ratio is required to clarify the presence of proteinuria, as if present, in combination with new-onset hypertension, would support the diagnosis of pre-eclampsia. The absence of proteinuria, however, does not exclude the diagnosis (see Table 8.2).

Urine toxicology screen as the use of recreational drugs, such as cocaine, can result in acute hypertension.

An ECG may identify left ventricular hypertrophy.

Chest radiography should be considered if pulmonary oedema or other pathology such as infection is suspected.

An echocardiogram to look for evidence of structural heart disease may also be helpful.

Renal ultrasound to look for underlying structural renal abnormalities is required, but the urgency of this depends on the clinical situation.

Cranial imaging with CT or MRI is not routinely required in all individuals with hypertension and headache, but should be arranged urgently if there are any specific neurological signs or symptoms suggestive of focal lesions such as haemorrhage, ischaemic stroke, or PRES.

Table 8.2 Definitions of hypertensive disorders of pregnancy

Gestational hypertension	New-onset hypertension after 20 weeks with no other features of pre-eclampsia
Pre-eclampsia	Hypertension after 20 weeks *AND* One or more of the following: • Proteinuria • Other maternal organ dysfunction, e.g. renal insufficiency (biochemical markers > the normal range in the absence of an alternative cause) • Utero-placental dysfunction (fetal growth restriction)
HELLP	Evidence of: • Haemolysis (elevated LDH, fragments on blood film, ↓ Hb) • Elevated liver enzymes • Low platelets

Reprinted from Collins S and Frise C. *Obstetric Medicine* (Oxford University Press, 2020) with permission from Oxford University Press.

3. Her blood pressure remains elevated despite the oral treatment, so what treatment would you give next?

The definition of high blood pressure requiring treatment in pregnancy is 140/ 90 mmHg or above. Now pregnancy has been identified, ramipril should be discontinued, and medications such as labetalol, modified-release nifedipine, or methyldopa are advised. Labetalol is licensed in pregnancy, safe and effective for managing hypertensive emergencies. This can be given orally or intravenously. A low threshold for intravenous therapy is recommended in severe hypertension or a hypertensive emergency (where target organ damage is occurring such as papilloedema, renal impairment, or neurological sequelae). There is no consensus for target blood pressure in the first few hours of therapy, but a reduction to a systolic blood pressure of 150–160 mmHg in the first 4–6 hours is suggested in women with very severe hypertension to avoid a precipitous drop in blood pressure risking a rapid reduction in cerebral and fetal perfusion. The target from then on is 135/ 85 mmHg or lower, in accordance with NICE Hypertension in Pregnancy guidelines.

4. Would you give her LMWH for VTE prophylaxis?

Pregnancy is a prothrombotic state so VTE prophylaxis should be considered in all hospitalized pregnant women. The presence of severe hypertension is a contra-indication to the use of LMWH. The initial uncertainty about pregnancy and whether delivery will be required is also a reason for taking a short time to establish more clinical information before LMWH is given.

She had an ultrasound that showed a single intrauterine pregnancy, with estimated fetal weight of 600 g. Gestation was estimated at 26 weeks and the baby was considered to be growth restricted.

Questions

5. What treatment does she require?
6. Does she need emergency delivery?
7. Does she need any additional assessment or tests?

Answers

5. What treatment does she require?

Antihypertensives should be prescribed to optimize blood pressure control and it is likely this will require a combination of oral agents.

Corticosteroids to aid fetal lung maturation should also be offered after discussion with the obstetric team about delivery timing.

Intravenous magnesium sulphate may be required for seizure prophylaxis if hypertension is not controlled or any features of severe pre-eclampsia emerge. Even if not used for this indication, it would also be offered at the time of preterm birth as this also provides some fetal neuroprotection.

6. Does she need emergency delivery?

Timing of birth for women with early-onset pre-eclampsia will depend on a balance between maternal and fetal health. At 26–28 weeks of gestation, the infant has a 30–60% chance of survival, but the risk of long-term morbidity is high. Survival and the chances of long-term sequelae of preterm birth improve with each additional week of gestation. On the other hand, continuing the pregnancy when severe placental dysfunction has developed risks intrauterine fetal death or abruption.

This patient already has emerging pre-eclampsia, given her symptoms, hypertension, and organ involvement (renal and liver impairment, low platelets). Urgent delivery planning is required. The maternal condition must be stabilized as far as possible before birth. At this gestation with the potential severity of fetal and maternal compromise, a caesarean birth would be required.

7. Does she need any additional assessment or tests?

There are certain conditions which predispose to early-onset pre-eclampsia that are important to consider, which include:

Chronic renal disease (check previous renal function, urine microscopy, renal ultrasound).

Antiphospholipid syndrome (consider postpartum measurement of lupus anticoagulant, anticardiolipin, and anti-B2 glycoprotein-1 antibodies).

Systemic lupus erythematosus (careful history and examination, FBC, urinalysis, ANA, ENA, and complement).

Conditions such as *thrombotic thrombocytopenic purpura* and *haemolytic uraemic syndrome*.

Chronic hypertension may be suspected at the time of this presentation, following the review of booking blood pressure or previous readings from primary/secondary care encounters, or it may become apparent when blood pressure does not entirely normalize in the weeks to months after delivery. Further tests that need to be considered in this setting include:

- Clinical examination for radioradial/radiofemoral delay, abdominal bruits
- Ambulatory blood pressure monitoring

- ECG +/– echocardiogram
- Bloods for potassium
- Renin:aldosterone ratio
- Overnight dexamethasone suppression test
- Urinary or plasma metanephrines for phaeochromocytoma
- Renal ultrasound
- MR angiogram renal arteries

Further reading

1. Hypertension in pregnancy: Diagnosis and management (NICE guideline NG133, 2019). <https://www.nice.org.uk/guidance/ng133>
2. Premature labour and birth. (NICE guideline NG25, updated 2019). <https://www.nice.org.uk/guidance/ng25>
3. **K. Duhig** *et al*. Placental growth factor testing to assess women with suspected pre-eclampsia: A multicentre, pragmatic, stepped-wedge cluster—randomised controlled trial. Lancet. 2019; **393**(10183): 1807–18.

Case 9

A 32-year-old woman presented to the Emergency Department with shortness of breath 3 weeks after the birth of her first child. The pregnancy had been uneventful, and she had an uncomplicated vaginal birth after spontaneous labour at 40 weeks of gestation. She was discharged the day following birth. She described worsening short of breath over the preceding week. This was worse on exertion, and she was unable to walk up the stairs. She also felt occasionally short of breath at rest. She did not wake up at night feeling breathless but was sleeping on four pillows as she felt short of breath lying any flatter. She had also noticed palpitations over the last 3 days but did not have any chest pain.

She had no other significant past medical history or family history. She was on no regular medications and did not smoke.

Initial assessment

General inspection:	Unwell, GCS 15/15
Heart rate:	120 bpm
Blood pressure:	110/70 mmHg
Respiratory rate:	22 breaths/min
Temperature:	36.4 °C
Oxygen saturations:	93% on room air
Urinalysis:	No protein

Examination

Cardiovascular:	Normal heart sounds, soft systolic murmur at apex
Respiratory:	Bilateral crackles at both bases
Abdomen:	Soft, non-tender abdomen, well contracted uterus
Legs:	Pitting oedema to knees

Bloods

See Table 9.1.

Table 9.1 Bloods

Haemoglobin	121 g/L
WCC	6.3×10^9/L
Platelets	203×10^9/L
Sodium	138 mmol/L
Potassium	3.9 mmol/L
Urea	3.8 mmol/L
Creatinine	35 µmol/L
Bilirubin	9 µmol/L
ALT	30 iU/L
Albumin	32 g/L
CRP	14 mg/L
D-dimer	1180 ng/mL
BNP	1615 pg/mL

Chest radiograph

See Figure 9.1.

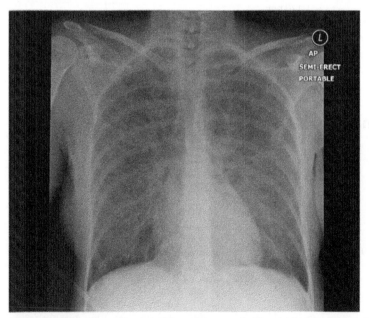

Figure 9.1 Chest X-ray. Reprinted from Adamson D, Dhanjal M, and Nelson-Piercy C (2011) *Heart Disease in Pregnancy*: Oxford University Press, with permission from Oxford University Press.

Questions

1. What are the possible causes for her symptoms?
2. Which investigations would you like to request?
3. How should this patient be treated?
4. Is bromocriptine treatment of potential benefit here?
5. What advice would you give her about future pregnancies?

Answers

1. What are the possible causes for her symptoms?

Peripartum cardiomyopathy (PPCM) is defined as heart failure that occurs at the end of pregnancy or in the months after birth with no other cause identified, and a left ventricular ejection fraction of less than 45%. It is rare, affecting 1 in 100–10,000 births and the cause is unknown. Risk factors for PPCM include older maternal age, Black or African heritage, multiparity, multiple pregnancy, family history, smoking, hypertension, pre-eclampsia, malnutrition, and prolonged use of tocolytics.

Dilated cardiomyopathy (DCM) may be inherited (several gene variants that cause DCM have been identified) or acquired (e.g. post-viral DCM). Women with DCM often have a significant deterioration in LV function during pregnancy. There is an increased risk of maternal mortality, especially with worse functional baseline (New York Heart Association class III or IV), ejection fraction less than 40%, mitral regurgitation, right ventricular failure, atrial fibrillation, and/or hypotension. Previously undiagnosed DCM which presents in pregnancy, particularly towards the end, can be difficult to distinguish from PPCM, so it is essential to take a thorough history to elicit any evidence of pre-existing heart disease or family history.

Ischaemic heart disease is a significant cause of maternal death, especially as the average age of pregnant women is increasing. Classical risk factors include hypertension, family history of ischaemic heart disease, cerebrovascular or vascular disease, pre-existing diabetes, smoking, and hypercholesterolaemia, but women can still get myocardial ischaemia in pregnancy and the postpartum period in the absence of these risk factors. Whilst thrombotic events can occur, coronary artery dissection occurs more commonly in pregnancy and postpartum compared to non-pregnant individuals. Chest pain is common in pregnant women with ischaemic heart disease, but the absence of chest pain does not exclude this diagnosis.

Hypertrophic cardiomyopathy is a pre-existing cardiomyopathy characterized by asymmetrical increase in myocardial thickness. Inheritance is autosomal dominant. Many women are asymptomatic, and these women usually tolerate pregnancy well. Approximately 30% of women overall have a worsening of symptoms in pregnancy. Women should be screened for arrhythmias, and beta-blockers continued if taken prior to conception.

Arrhythmias when poorly tolerated or persistent, including atrial tachycardias and atrial fibrillation, or even a heavy burden of ventricular ectopy, may cause impaired LV function and the symptoms of heart failure. An ECG and/or ambulatory monitoring is crucial for identifying an underlying arrhythmia.

Pulmonary embolism risk is high in pregnancy and postpartum. Pulmonary emboli do not cause signs of left ventricular impairment (i.e. pulmonary oedema), but significant clot burden can cause right heart failure, which may result in arrhythmias and symptoms such as peripheral oedema.

Takotsubo syndrome is an acute and typically reversible cause of heart failure. It appears to be triggered by emotional stress and is characterized by significant apical cardiac akinesia which causes severe but reversible left ventricular dysfunction.

2. What investigations should be requested?

An ECG is an essential investigation in any women where cardiac disease is a possibility. A normal ECG is very reassuring and reduces the likelihood that a subsequent echocardiogram will be abnormal. The ECG in women with PPCM is rarely normal, and tachycardia is a predictor of poor outcome.

Chest radiography is required in all women with significant shortness of breath and may show pulmonary oedema and/or pleural effusions in those with heart failure. If there is concern about pulmonary emboli, cross-sectional imaging with computed tomography or ventilation/perfusion scanning should also be performed.

Echocardiography should be performed as soon as possible in women with signs or symptoms suggestive of heart failure in pregnancy or postpartum and will help to clarify the underlying diagnosis.

Natriuretic peptides (BNP or pro-NT-BNP) are normal or only slightly increased above the non-pregnant baseline in pregnancy. A significant rise above the normal range is indicative of cardiac disease, and serial measurements can be used to monitor disease progress and response to treatment.

Cardiac MRI is an excellent imaging modality for providing further clarification about the nature of a cardiomyopathy. The use of gadolinium contrast is usually avoided in pregnancy if possible, so often it is appropriate to delay a cardiac MRI until after birth.

3. How would you treat this woman?

Urgent assessment is required to determine the severity of the heart failure, as well as the appropriate immediate management and location of ongoing care.

Treatments that can be used in pregnancy or the postpartum period include:

- Loop diuretics
- Beta-blockers
- Aspirin
- Nitrates
- Hydralazine
- LMWH (dose depends on clinical situation)

Medication that is only used after birth:

- ACE inhibitors (captopril or enalapril are preferred if breastfeeding)
- Ivabradine (usually avoided in breastfeeding)
- Mineralocorticoid receptor antagonists

Women who are in cardiogenic shock or severe heart failure should be referred to a specialist centre and reviewed by a multidisciplinary team including cardiologists, intensivists, obstetricians, neonatologists, anaesthetists, and possibly cardiac surgeons. Women may require inotropes, invasive or non-invasive ventilation, mechanical circulatory assistance, left ventricular assist devices, or extra-corporeal membrane oxygenation.

4. Is bromocriptine treatment of potential benefit here?

This is a disputed area of peripartum cardiomyopathy treatment. There is evidence that a cleaved form of prolactin is proapoptotic and worsens cardiac function. A limited number of studies have suggested that bromocriptine improves outcome in women with peripartum cardiomyopathy. The role of bromocriptine, and stopping breastfeeding, should be discussed with women with peripartum cardiomyopathy.

5. What advice would you give her about future pregnancies?

All women should remain on treatment for 12–24 months and therefore discussion about effective contraception is a priority. Counselling about future pregnancy is very important and the prognosis in a future pregnancy depends on how well cardiac function recovers following the affected pregnancy:

- If LVEF returns to over 50%, then while there is a risk of relapse, there is a very low risk of heart failure or death.
- If LVEF remains under 50%, then a future pregnancy is associated with a high risk of relapse, and a risk of heart failure and death. There is also a risk of preterm birth and fetal death.
- If LVEF is under 30%, then pregnancy should be discouraged.

Further reading

1. J. Bauersachs *et al.* Pathophysiology, diagnosis and management of peripartum cardiomyopathy: A position statement from the Heart Failure Association of the European Society of Cardiology Study Group on peripartum cardiomyopathy. European Journal of Heart Failure. 2019; **21**: 827–43.
2. K. Sliwa *et al.* Long-term prognosis, subsequent pregnancy, contraception and overall management of peripartum cardiomyopathy: practical guidance paper from the Heart Failure Association of the European Society of Cardiology Study Group on Peripartum Cardiomyopathy. European Journal of Heart Failure, 2018; **20**: 951–62.
3. K. Sliwa *et al.* Risk stratification and management of women with cardiomyopathy/heart failure planning pregnancy or presenting during/after pregnancy: a position statement from the Heart Failure Association of the European Society of Cardiology Study Group on Peripartum Cardiomyopathy. European Journal of Heart Failure. 2021; **23**(4): 527–540.

Case 10

A 25-year-old woman had a history of renal disease secondary to focal segmental glomerulosclerosis and was having regular haemodialysis via tunnelled catheter. She had been on the transplant list for a year, but no match had been identified. She attended the Emergency Department with abdominal pain, fever, vomiting, and concern about sepsis. She still passed small volumes of urine and did not have any symptoms of urine infection.

She had no other past medical history. She was taking alfacalcidol three times a week, erythropoietin injections twice a week, ramipril daily, and intermittently received intravenous iron whilst on haemodialysis. She had no family history of any illnesses and had never smoked.

Initial assessment

General inspection:	Unwell, dehydrated
Heart rate:	125 bpm
Blood pressure:	88/56 mmHg
Respiratory rate:	20 breaths/min
Temperature:	38.2 °C
Oxygen saturations:	99% on room air
Urinalysis:	3+ protein, 3+ ketones
	HCG positive

Examination

Cardiovascular:	Normal heart sounds, no murmurs
Respiratory:	Normal breath sounds
Abdomen:	Right iliac fossa tenderness
Line site:	No evidence of erythema surrounding line insertion site
Throat:	Normal

Bloods

See Table 10.1.

Table 10.1 Bloods

Haemoglobin	102 g/L
WCC	14.1 × 10⁹/L
Platelets	220 × 10⁹/L
Sodium	134 mmol/L
Potassium	5.4 mmol/L
Urea	20.2 mmol/L
Creatinine	415 µmol/L
Bilirubin	4 µmol/L
ALT	30 iU/L
ALP	60 iU/L
Albumin	27 g/L
CRP	109 mg/L
Amylase	50 U/L

Questions

1. What are the potential causes for this presentation?
2. What other investigations would you like to perform?
3. What are the management priorities for this woman?
4. What are the implications of chronic kidney disease for pregnancy?

Answers

1. What are the potential causes for this presentation?

Ectopic pregnancy should always be considered in a woman of reproductive age with a positive pregnancy test and abdominal pain. Pain can be localized to either lower quadrant, be generalized (suggesting significant abdominal bleeding) or be felt in the shoulder tip/supraclavicular region (referred pain as a result of phrenic nerve activation by blood in contact with the diaphragmatic peritoneum). Vaginal bleeding is variably present, but other symptoms include loose stool, vomiting, and maternal collapse.

Acute appendicitis should always be considered when abdominal pain occurs, the classical location for which is the right iliac fossa, but pain can be atypical particularly in later pregnancy.

Miscarriage causes intermittent cramping lower abdominal pain with or without vaginal bleeding. If there is fever then *septic miscarriage* would be suspected, which can be spontaneous but is more likely to be a complication of an incomplete spontaneous miscarriage or pregnancy termination.

Pelvic inflammatory disease usually occurs secondary to sexually transmitted infections, most commonly *Chlamydia trachomatis* or *Neisseria gonorrhoea* but can arise from normal vaginal flora e.g. *Gardnerella sp.* Symptoms include acute abdominal pain, fever, and vomiting. Right hypochondrial and shoulder pain may also feature (Fitz-Hugh–Curtis syndrome). Ascending genital tract infection may cause a tubo-ovarian abscess. A thorough sexual history should be established. On examination there may be cervical motion tenderness.

Ovarian pathologies including ruptured ovarian cysts or ovarian torsion may cause acute pain and vomiting.

Urinary tract infection and/or pyelonephritis must be considered with this presentation. Blood cultures and a mid-stream urine sample for culture should ideally be taken prior to administration of any antibiotics.

Renal colic presents with severe spasmodic abdominal pain which can radiate classically from 'loin to groin'. If there are signs of infection, then an infected obstructed kidney is a possibility, which requires urgent imaging and treatment (insertion of a nephrostomy).

2. What other investigations would you like to perform?

Imaging

Bedside Focused Assessment with Sonography in Trauma (FAST) ultrasound can be performed by suitably trained staff and will exclude major abdominal bleeding.

Abdominal ultrasound is easy to obtain and may identify renal or appendiceal pathology.

Pelvic ultrasound is best performed by the transvaginal route and is mandatory to identify the location of the pregnancy. This study is also suited for the identification of ovarian, tubal and uterine abnormalities.

Cross-sectional imaging (CT/MRI) may be required. Due to the fetal dose of radiation from abdominal CT imaging this is often avoided, and MRI used in preference.

Bloods

Serum HCG measurement is not required routinely when a urinary HCG is found to be positive at the time of an acute presentation. Its role is in serial testing for a *pregnancy of unknown location*, or in monitoring of a confirmed ectopic pregnancy.

Microbiology

- Mid-stream urine for culture
- Blood cultures
- Line cultures
- High vaginal swab for MC&S
- Vaginal or urinary swabs should be obtained for *Chlamydia* and *N. gonorrhoea* nucleic acid amplification testing

3. What are the management priorities for this woman?

Treatment of infection

She requires broad spectrum antibiotics, prescribed according to local antimicrobial prescribing policies for individuals requiring renal replacement therapy. These can then be rationalized when culture results are available.

Fluid balance

Whilst she passes small volumes of urine, her kidney disease means that she is at risk of fluid overload and therefore small volume boluses are required if intravenous fluids are indicated because of concern about sepsis and hypotension. Daily weight is a useful indicator of fluid balance as she will be aware of her 'dry weight' as this is recorded when on haemodialysis.

Discussion about pregnancy continuation

If there is a viable pregnancy present on the pelvic US, then she requires early discussion about the risks of remaining pregnant, as well as the options available to her which include termination of pregnancy. She is on the transplant list, so if she were to have a successful renal transplant, a pregnancy after that would be associated with fewer pregnancy complications.

Pregnancy specifics

She should be started on daily folic acid supplements, which should be 5 mg daily due to increased loss of water-soluble vitamins whilst on haemodialysis.

Blood pressure

Her ACE inhibitor should be discontinued and replaced with an alternative antihypertensive if this is being used for hypertension (rather than solely for proteinuria). The use of a maternity early warning score is advised in all pregnant women, but this may not be common practice if the patient is on a medical or gynaecology ward rather than an obstetric setting given the early gestation. It is therefore important to ensure that these are used when her observations are measured, or the responsible team are aware of the relevant blood pressure thresholds used in pregnant women.

VTE prophylaxis

If she has nephrotic-range proteinuria, then LMWH prophylaxis is advised. In practice this is a weight-based dose (that does not require adjustment with renal function) but is only given on non-dialysis days, due to the administration of anticoagulation whilst receiving dialysis.

Aspirin

She requires low-dose aspirin prophylaxis from 12 weeks of gestation given the risk of pre-eclampsia and intrauterine growth restriction.

4. What are the implications of chronic kidney disease for pregnancy?

CKD is associated with a variety of adverse pregnancy outcomes, the incidence of which increases with the degree of renal impairment. Fetal risks include growth restriction, stillbirth, and preterm birth. The implications of prematurity and extended neonatal ITU admission are also important considerations and it is important to include these when counselling women with CKD. Maternal risks include miscarriage, pre-eclampsia (which can develop at an early gestation), venous thromboembolism, and a deterioration in renal function. This can be significant and in women with advanced CKD, pregnancy hastens the time to renal replacement therapy being required.

In women not yet requiring haemodialysis, this may be required during pregnancy for fetal or maternal indications, including concerns about high urea and fetotoxicity in the former, or management of electrolytes, fluid balance, or acid/base in the latter. If haemodialysis is commenced, there is a possibility that women are left dialysis-dependent after birth.

Even if haemodialysis is not required in pregnancy, the renal function of women with CKD often takes a step down in pregnancy, which may recover after birth but will persist in some women.

Women established on haemodialysis are advised to increase their number of hours on dialysis from early in pregnancy as this has been shown to improve pregnancy outcomes. This can be increased gradually to allow increased tolerability of the fluid shifts, aiming for around 36 hours per week. Haemodialysis targets take account of weight and electrolyte fluctuations, based on the woman's dry weight, which will increase as pregnancy progresses. The aim is to optimize the maternal biochemistry as much as possible. Additional phosphate in the dialysate and increased erythropoietin supplementation may also be required.

Further reading

1. **K. Wiles** *et al.* The Renal Association clinical practice guideline pregnancy and renal disease. 2019. <https://ukkidney.org/sites/renal.org/files/FINAL-Pregnancy-Guideline-September-2019.pdf>

Case 11

A 44-year-old woman attended for pre-conception counselling following a review in the local fertility service. She had been trying to conceive with her current partner for four years. She had had two first trimester miscarriages during this time. Past medical history was notable for polycystic ovarian syndrome, with six to eight spontaneous periods each year. She takes metformin 500 mg twice daily as well as pregnancy multivitamins. She is a non-smoker and drinks approximately 15 units of alcohol per week.

The fertility service asked for advice about her thyroid function.

Bloods

See Table 11.1.

Table 11.1 Bloods

TSH	3.5 mIU/l
fT4	18.6 pmol/l
fT3	4.7 pmol/l
TPO antibody	positive

Questions

1. What treatment for her thyroid would you suggest while she is undergoing fertility treatment?
2. What is overt hypothyroidism, what implications does it have for pregnancy and how is it treated?
3. What is subclinical hypothyroidism and how is it treated in pregnancy?
4. What is isolated hypothyroxinaemia and how is it managed in pregnancy?
5. The patient has found some thyroid products online which claim to be of benefit, what do you advise her?

Answers

1. What treatment would you suggest while she is undergoing fertility treatment?

No specific treatment is required for this woman's thyroid function tests. Though she is TPO antibody positive, she is euthyroid.

TPO antibody positivity in euthyroid women has been associated with an increased rate of miscarriage compared to women who are TPO antibody negative. Large multicentre studies have, however, not shown improvement in live birth rates if these women are treated with thyroxine. These women are also at increased risk of developing overt hypothyroidism. Regular monitoring of thyroid function is therefore appropriate while she is trying to conceive and in pregnancy. Women who are TPO antibody positive are also at increased risk of postpartum thyroiditis, so thyroid function should also be checked 3 months postpartum.

2. What is overt hypothyroidism, what implications does it have for pregnancy and how is it treated?

According to the American Thyroid Association (ATA) 2017 guidelines for the 'Diagnosis and Management of Thyroid Disease during Pregnancy and the Postpartum', overt hypothyroidism in pregnancy is defined as a TSH greater than 10 mIU/l associated with a fT4 of any level OR a TSH over the upper limit of trimester-specific reference range (or over 4.0 mIU/l in the absence of local reference ranges) and fT4 below the lower limit of the trimester-specific reference range. This is associated with an increased risk of miscarriage and pre-eclampsia, as well as premature birth, low birth weight, and impaired neurological development. This should be treated with levothyroxine, aiming for a TSH within the trimester-specific reference ranges. It is well known that the normal ranges for thyroid biochemistry are different in pregnancy, however the exact range depends on the assay and therefore it is recommended that local reference ranges are used if available.

In women treated with levothyroxine prior to pregnancy, thyroid function tests should be checked urgently once pregnancy is confirmed and levothyroxine dose adjusted if required. If urgent testing is not possible, women should be advised to increase their levothyroxine dose by about 30% and have thyroid function tests checked soon. It is important for women to be careful about dose timings, to avoid taking their thyroxine at a similar time of day to other medications, foods or drinks such as tea, all of which may affect thyroxine absorption.

3. What is subclinical hypothyroidism and how is it managed in pregnancy?

Subclinical hypothyroidism is defined in the ATA 2017 guidelines as a TSH greater than the upper limit of trimester-specific reference range but less than 10 mIU/l, alongside a fT4 within the normal range. Evidence is inconsistent about the effect of subclinical hypothyroidism on the risk of miscarriage, hypertension, pre-eclampsia, or fetal growth and development. However, there is no evidence that treatment of subclinical hypothyroidism with levothyroxine improves maternal or fetal outcomes. There is no evidence that treatment improves childhood IQ, though all studies started treatment at the end of the first trimester or later. Nevertheless, treatment seems prudent if TSH is elevated above the upper limit of trimester-specific reference ranges and the woman is TPO antibody positive, as this combination does appear to be particularly related to an increased risk of first trimester miscarriage.

4. What is isolated hypothyroxinaemia and how is it managed in pregnancy?

In isolated hypothyroxinaemia the TSH is within the normal limit, but fT4 is below the trimester-specific reference range. It is associated with a raised BMI, as well as iodine deficiency and excess. Isolated hypothyroxinaemia has an impact on fetal neurodevelopment, with a reduction in childhood IQ. There is no evidence, however, that treatment improves outcomes.

5. The patient has found some thyroid products online which claim to be of benefit, what do you advise her?

A range of thyroid products are available to purchase, for example desiccated porcine thyroid extract, and are often marketed as 'natural' thyroid replacement. These are not recommended in pregnancy. In particular, women should avoid using compounds containing T3, either desiccated thyroid or compound T3/T4 preparations. Treatment with T3 leads to a relatively low maternal T4 level. T4 is crucial for the developing fetal brain, particularly in early pregnancy. T3 does not cross readily into the fetal central nervous system, so therefore only levothyroxine treatment should be advocated in pregnancy.

Table 11.2 Thyroid disease during pregnancy

	TSH	fT4	Maternal and fetal consequences	Treatment
Overt hypothyroidism	Above 10 mIU/l OR Above trimester-specific normal range (or > 4 mIU/l)	Any level Below trimester-specific normal range	Increased risk of miscarriage, preterm birth, low birth weight, impaired neurological development	Levothyroxine
Subclinical hypothyroidism	Above trimester specific normal range (or > 4 mIU/l) but below 10 mIU/l	Within trimester specific normal range	Possible effect on miscarriage, hypertension, pre-eclampsia, fetal growth and development.	Can be considered in women who are TPO antibody positive
Isolated hypo-thyroxinaemia	Within trimester-specific normal range	Below trimester specific normal range	Impaired fetal neurodevelopment	Ensure sufficient iodine supplementation

Further reading

1. **R. Dhillon-Smith** *et al*. Levothyroxine in women with thyroid peroxidase antibodies before conception. New England Journal of Medicine. 2019; **380**:1316–25.
2. T. **Korevaar** *et al*. Thyroid disease in pregnancy: New insights in diagnosis and clinical management. Nature Reviews Endocrinology. 2017; **13**: 610–22.
3. **E. Alexander** *et al*. 2017 Guidelines of the American Thyroid Association for the diagnosis and management of thyroid disease during pregnancy and the postpartum. Thyroid. 2017; **27**(3): 315–89. <https://www.liebertpub.com/doi/10.1089/thy.2016.0457>

Case 12

A 20-year-old woman presented at 28 weeks of gestation in her first pregnancy with a 2-week history of palpitations. They were occurring daily, lasting for 10–15 minutes, and usually occurred at rest. There was no associated chest pain, shortness of breath, or syncope. She had had no previous episodes and was otherwise fit and well, with no significant past medical history. She was not on any regular medication, and she had never smoked. Her booking BP was 100/70 mmHg and BMI was 24 kg/m².

Initial assessment

General inspection: Looks well
Heart rate: 110 bpm
Blood pressure: 90/60 mmHg
Respiratory rate: 16 breaths/min
Temperature: 36.2 °C
Oxygen saturations: 99% on room air
Urinalysis: No protein

Examination

Cardiovascular: Normal heart sounds, no murmurs
Respiratory: Normal breath sounds
Abdomen: Soft abdomen, non-tender gravid uterus

Bloods

See Table 12.1.

Table 12.1 Bloods

Haemoglobin	107 g/L
WCC	7.2×10^9/L
Platelets	255×10^9/L
Sodium	138 mmol/L
Potassium	4.7 mmol/L
Urea	2.1 mmol/L
Creatinine	38 µmol/L
Bilirubin	4 µmol/L
ALT	6 iU/L
ALP	68 iU/L
Albumin	28 g/L

Questions

1. At what level of heart rate should clinicians be concerned?
2. What are the potential causes for her symptoms?
3. What other investigations would you like to perform?
4. How would you treat her?
5. What adjustments at delivery are required?

Answers

1. At what level of heart rate should clinicians be concerned?

It has long been recognized that pregnancy leads to an increase in resting maternal heart rate. This was historically described as an increase in 10–20 bpm, with the acceptance of a slightly higher upper limit in a woman with a higher BMI. However, more recent data have shown that the normal range of heart rate in pregnancy encompasses a wider range than that suggested previously, and that heart rates of more than 100 bpm were common (more than 10% of observations taken in early pregnancy), as were heart rates of more than 105 bpm from 28 weeks. With this recent evaluation of physiological parameters in pregnancy, an absolute value for the upper limit of normal in pregnancy is difficult to define. A cut-off value of 100 bpm will be too low for many women, resulting in over-investigation, whilst 120 bpm is likely to be too high, resulting in false reassurance and the potential to miss clinically important diagnoses. The MBRRACE-UK 2015–2017 report recommends that 'a persistent sinus tachycardia is a "red flag" and should always be investigated, particularly when there are associated symptoms i.e. breathlessness'.

2. What are the potential causes for her symptoms?

Secondary sinus tachycardia

The concern reflected in the MBRRACE-UK recommendation is the result of the fact that a sinus tachycardia can occur in many other conditions, most concerningly haemorrhage (concealed abruption or unrecognized postpartum haemorrhage), pulmonary emboli, and sepsis. A sinus tachycardia can also result from pain or dehydration. However, pregnant women may often look very well, and this may be the only abnormality in their observations, which then may result in this being put aside when other tests are normal.

Pulmonary emboli can often present with palpitations, and a sinus tachycardia is often seen in women with pulmonary emboli. However, there are many women with a sinus tachycardia that do not have pulmonary emboli, and therefore do not require investigation for this. A careful history is required for other symptoms that might point towards this diagnosis. Risk stratification tools and criteria to rule out pulmonary emboli based on biomarkers such as D-dimer are not validated in pregnancy, therefore it is advised that these are not used in the assessment of pregnant women with a possible PE.

Infection can manifest with a sinus tachycardia as the first objective abnormality and a thorough history and examination is required to look for a possible source of infection.

Anaemia is common in pregnancy and can result in both a tachycardia and symptoms such as palpitations and/or breathlessness.

Hyperthyroidism is an uncommon cause of palpitations in pregnancy, but any woman presenting with this should be asked about potential symptoms of hyperthyroidism and have their thyroid function checked.

Lifestyle contributors should also be considered, including caffeine intake. Medications such as salbutamol inhalers can cause a tachycardia, so a careful medication history is important.

Rhythm abnormalities

Ectopic beats are not always an abnormal finding, but they may cause symptoms in pregnancy, perhaps because of an increase in frequency but also potentially a result of the increase of cardiac output making these feel more prominent when they occur. A classical history of infrequent ectopy does not require further investigation, but if the symptoms are prominent and frequent, then concern arises about a high ectopy 'burden' (above 10%), which can result in left ventricular dysfunction and cardiomyopathy. In this situation, ambulatory monitoring is recommended and consideration of echocardiogram and treatment depending on the findings.

Inappropriate sinus tachycardia accounts for a significant number of pregnant women with a tachycardia. Episodes of sinus tachycardia may be confirmed on ambulatory monitoring, and this can be diagnosed if the women are otherwise well and no underlying cause for the tachycardia is identified.

Narrow complex tachycardias

Supraventricular tachycardia includes AV-re-entrant tachycardia (AVRT) and AV-nodal re-entrant tachycardia (AVNRT). AVRT occurs when the re-entry circuit is caused by accessory pathways, as opposed to AVNRT, which occurs when the re-entry circuit involves the AV node. P waves are therefore present (but can be atypical) on an ECG of an individual with AVNRT, but absent in someone with AVRT. The management of these includes vagal manoeuvres, pharmacological agents (adenosine, beta-blockers, calcium channel blockers such as verapamil), and interventional techniques, such as catheter ablation of the accessory pathway. Amiodarone is usually avoided in pregnancy due to effects on the fetal thyroid.

Atrial tachycardia is uncommon in pregnancy but can be mistaken for a sinus tachycardia. The ECG in an atrial tachycardia shows an atrial rate generally greater than 100 bpm and abnormal p waves, which may be inverted or biphasic. Ambulatory ECG monitoring may aid diagnosis as a sinus tachycardia will wax and wane, and reduce overnight, whereas an atrial tachycardia will show a more consistent elevation in rate.

Atrial fibrillation and atrial flutter are uncommon in pregnancy, and historically have been associated with underlying structural heart disease. More recent data suggest this pattern is not so clear cut, and it can occur in women with no structural heart disease. Atrial fibrillation is characterized by chaotic and disorganized atrial activity, demonstrated by absent p waves on the ECG and an irregularly irregular rhythm. Atrial flutter is caused by a re-entry circuit in the right atrium, with organized atrial activity. The ECG characteristically shows a 'saw-tooth' pattern, with a regular atrial rate of between 200 and 400 bpm.

Broad complex tachycardias

Ventricular tachycardia is a rare cause of palpitations in pregnancy and is an unlikely cause of an isolated tachycardia in an otherwise well individual. The presence of structural heart disease increases the chance of this occurring so the coexistence of palpitations or tachycardia in these women should be urgently investigated. It can be monomorphic or polymorphic, and can occur in association with long QT syndrome, Brugada syndrome, and hypertrophic cardiomyopathy. If this occurs only in pregnancy, there is a high likelihood that it will resolve after birth.

3. What other investigations would you like to perform?

A careful history and examination are required in all women with palpitations and/or a tachycardia, with consideration of the following tests to help clarify the underlying diagnosis.

An ECG is the most important investigation, as if this is performed at the time of an episode of palpitations or tachycardia and confirms a rhythm abnormality, other investigations may not be required. If the ECG shows sinus rhythm when the patient is tachycardic or symptomatic, then an additional rhythm disturbance is unlikely.

Bloods including a FBC, electrolytes, thyroid function, and CRP, with blood cultures also if infection is suspected.

Further diagnostic tests

Echocardiography aids the identification of structural heart disease, as well as assessment of left ventricular function in the setting of a tachycardia. This is not necessarily required in all women with palpitations or a mild sinus tachycardia but would be recommended if there was any suspicion of structural heart disease or compromise from an underlying abnormal rhythm.

Ambulatory monitoring can be performed for 24–48 hours or for a longer period such as 5 to 7 days, depending on the reported frequency of events. This may show the nature of rhythm at time of symptoms, as well as the burden of ectopic beats.

An implantable loop recorder is less relevant for women with an ongoing tachycardia but can be used if women have significant symptoms but infrequently (e.g. a single collapse with significant consequences and high suspicion of cardiac arrhythmia) as this recorder can be implanted for several months.

Imaging for pulmonary emboli is required if there are other symptoms that suggest underlying PE may be present.

4. How would you treat her?

The most likely diagnosis is an inappropriate sinus tachycardia if other investigations are all reassuring. Medical treatment is therefore not required, but these women often benefit from advice about potential contributors such as caffeine, and reassurance that this arrhythmia whilst annoying if symptoms are prominent, is not concerning.

Infrequently, beta-blockade with bisoprolol or metoprolol may be prescribed to those women with frequent and/or very symptomatic palpitations. Observational studies have associated beta-blocker use with fetal growth restriction; however this may be confounded by the underlying conditions being treated in these cohorts, furthermore the absolute reduction in recorded birth weight was small. If a woman is taking regular beta-blockers for most of the pregnancy, serial third trimester growth scans may be warranted.

5. What adjustments at delivery are required?

An inappropriate or secondary tachycardia does not increase the risk of complications at the time of birth, however if this is prominent, birth would be preferable in a location where cardiac monitoring can be performed if required. A caesarean delivery is not required for management of a maternal arrhythmia. The presence of a baseline maternal tachycardia will make identification of true complications of labour and delivery harder, so careful attention should be paid to other symptoms and vital signs.

Further reading

1. **L. Green** *et al*. Gestation-specific vital sign reference ranges in pregnancy. Obstetrics & Gynecology. 2020; **135**: 653–64.
2. MBRRACE-UK Maternal Report 2019. Saving Lives, Improving Mothers' Care: Lessons learned to inform maternity care from the UK and Ireland Confidential Enquiries into Maternal Deaths and Morbidity 2015–17. <https://www.npeu.ox.ac.uk/assets/downloads/mbrr ace-uk/reports/MBRRACE-UK%20Maternal%20Report%202019%20-%20WEB%20VERS ION.pdf>

Case 13

A 39-year-old woman presented at 34 weeks of gestation with a tonic-clonic seizure. She had noticed a headache in the preceding few days. This was her first pregnancy, and her booking blood pressure had been 100/70 mmHg with a booking BMI of 23.5 kg/m². There was no history of previous seizures, head injury, or high blood pressure. She had no past medical history and had never smoked. Her family history included hypertension in both her mother and sister.

Initial assessment

General inspection:	Drowsy, responsive to voice and pain
Heart rate:	112 bpm
Blood pressure:	175/105 mmHg
Respiratory rate:	18 breaths/min
Temperature:	36.6 °C
Oxygen saturations:	99% on room air
Urinalysis:	2+ protein

Examination

Cardiovascular:	Normal heart sounds, no murmurs
Respiratory:	Normal breath sounds
Abdomen:	Mild epigastric tenderness; no peritonism; normal bowel sounds
	Gravid uterus appropriate size for dates
Neurology:	GCS 12 (E4, M5, V3)
	Normal tone, power, and sensation of upper and lower limbs
	Hyperreflexic with 5 beats of clonus
CTG:	Normal

Bloods

See Table 13.1.

Table 13.1 Bloods

Haemoglobin	99 g/L
WCC	10.7×10^9/L
Platelets	118×10^9/L
Sodium	138 mmol/L
Potassium	4.5 mmol/L
Urea	5.2 mmol/L
Creatinine	100 µmol/L
Bilirubin	28 µmol/L
ALT	30 iU/L
Albumin	27g/L
CRP	7 mg/L
Urate	380 µmol/L
LDH	1600 U/L
PT	14 s
APTT	30 s
Fibrinogen	4.0 g/L
Blood film	No red cell fragments, polychromasia

Questions

1. What is the most likely diagnosis?
2. What are the potential causes of a first seizure in a pregnant woman?
3. What investigations would you arrange?
4. What treatment would you initiate?
5. What postnatal complications are important to anticipate?

Answers

1. What is the most likely diagnosis?

The main abnormalities shown on the blood tests are anaemia, thrombocytopenia, and a possibility of haemolysis (high LDH) alongside normal coagulation parameters. She also has an acute kidney injury. The most likely diagnosis given the symptoms and haematological abnormalities is eclampsia, a tonic-clonic seizure in the setting of pregnancy-related hypertension.

2. What are the potential causes of a first seizure in a pregnant woman?

Metabolic causes such as hypoglycaemia or hyponatraemia can cause seizures, and as in non-pregnant individuals, venous sinus thrombosis, space-occupying lesions, and intracranial haemorrhage should be considered. Less common causes such as thrombotic thrombocytopenic purpura (TTP) can occur for the first time in pregnancy. The clinical features of this overlap with the symptoms and signs of pre-eclampsia so it can be difficult to distinguish. Epilepsy is a condition of repeated seizures, so whilst a first presentation of epilepsy in pregnancy is possible, this is less likely and a diagnosis of exclusion.

3. What investigations would you arrange?

Blood tests are essential; glucose and electrolytes are needed urgently. Blood tests looking to further clarify the degree of haemolysis are also required (reticulocyte count and direct antibody test in addition to the blood film and LDH already mentioned). ADAMTS13 level should be considered as, if low, this would be consistent with TTP.

Imaging such as CT head or MRI head should be considered if neurological abnormalities persist, or if the clinical situation does not clearly support a diagnosis of eclampsia. Plans for this should take into consideration practicalities such as the location of the patient and whether transfer for imaging is appropriate and safe.

A renal ultrasound may also be useful to see if there are any structural abnormalities contributing to the renal impairment.

4. What treatment would you initiate?

She requires antihypertensive treatment, which needs to be given intravenously if she is unable to take oral medication. Intravenous magnesium sulphate is also recommended for neuroprotection and reduces the chances of a further seizure occurring. Caution is required due to her acute kidney injury, as reduced renal clearance of magnesium increases the risk of toxicity. Steroids for fetal lung maturation should also be discussed given delivery is likely to be imminent. Fluid restriction to 80–85 ml/hr is also advisable in all women with eclampsia or severe pre-eclampsia. If further seizures occur, then a further bolus of magnesium sulphate, and treatment with intravenous levetiracetam, as well as intubation and ventilation should be considered and discussed with a senior multidisciplinary team.

She requires urgent delivery but only once her clinical condition is sufficiently stabilized (even if there is acute fetal compromise, maternal safety must remain the priority). Mode of birth would be emergency caesarean delivery unless she was already in labour and timely birth is expected. If the platelet count continues to drop, a general anaesthetic would be considered. Close liaison with the Haematology service is essential to ensure that blood products are available, including platelets and coagulation factors, as these may be required if she deteriorates further.

5. What postnatal complications are important to anticipate?

The effects of pre-eclampsia or eclampsia persist for several days after delivery. Hypertension may worsen before it improves, typically about 5 days after delivery. Alternative antihypertensives can be used when breastfeeding, including atenolol rather than labetalol, amlodipine rather than modified release nifedipine, and the ACE inhibitors captopril and enalapril. Methyldopa should be discontinued after delivery if used in pregnancy and replaced with an alternative.

Acute kidney injury can commonly worsen after delivery, to which bleeding at delivery may contribute; however renal replacement therapy is rarely required in women with hypertensive disorders of pregnancy.

Further reading

1. NICE. Hypertension in pregnancy: Diagnosis and management (NICE guideline No 133, 2019). <https://www.nice.org.uk/guidance/ng133>

Case 14

A 40-year-old woman in her first pregnancy with no past medical history presented at 35 weeks of gestation with a 3-day history of a sore throat. She had not been able to eat or drink anything for 24 hours and had also intermittently vomited. She did not report diarrhoea and no other family members were unwell. She had been entirely well until this point in her pregnancy, with normal blood pressure and BMI at booking. She was not on any medications. She was a non-smoker and did not drink alcohol.

Initial assessment

General inspection: Unwell, dehydrated
Heart rate: 110 bpm
Blood pressure: 90/60 mmHg
Respiratory rate: 40 breaths/min
Temperature: 36.8 °C
Oxygen saturations: 98% on room air
Urinalysis: No protein, 4+ ketones

Examination

Cardiovascular: Normal heart sounds, no murmurs
Respiratory: Normal breath sounds
Abdomen: Mild epigastric tenderness, no peritonism, normal bowel sounds
Throat: Erythematous tonsils with purulent exudate
Neck: Tender submandibular lymphadenopathy

Bloods

See Table 14.1.

Over the next 24 hours, she continued to vomit profusely and became increasingly unwell and tachycardic. Urinalysis again showed 4+ ketones.

Additional blood tests

See Table 14.2.

Table 14.1 Bloods

Haemoglobin	133 g/L
WCC	16.7 × 10⁹/L
Platelets	248 × 10⁹/L
Sodium	136 mmol/L
Potassium	4.0 mmol/L
Urea	5.2 mmol/L
Creatinine	79 μmol/L
Bilirubin	8 μmol/L
ALT	59 iU/L
ALP	100 iU/L
Albumin	28 g/L
CRP	154 mg/L
Amylase	50 U/L
Urate	450 μmol/L

Table 14.2 Additional blood tests

Capillary glucose	3.1 mmol/L
Capillary ketones	4.5 mmol/L

Arterial blood gas

See Table 14.3.

Table 14.3 Arterial blood gas

pH	7.29
PaCO$_2$	2.7 kPa
PaO$_2$	10.1 kPa
HCO$_3$	10.7 mmol/L
Base excess	−14.4 mmol/L
Chloride	110 mmol/L
Lactate	0.7 mmol/L

Questions

1. What metabolic derangement is shown here?
2. What are the differential diagnoses of the metabolic derangement?
3. Why is this metabolic derangement more common in pregnancy?
4. What is the likely underlying cause?
5. What investigations would you arrange?
6. How would you manage this woman?

Answers

1. What metabolic derangement is shown here?

The arterial blood gas results show a metabolic acidosis with partial respiratory compensation. The anion gap is elevated at 19.3 mmol/L (calculated as anion gap = (sodium + potassium) – (bicarbonate + chloride)) as the normal range is 12–16 mmol/L.

2. What are the differential diagnoses of the metabolic derangement?

Metabolic acidosis with an elevated anion gap occurs as a result of the accumulation of organic acids or impaired hydrogen ion secretion. Causes of a metabolic acidosis with an elevated anion gap include uraemia, lactic acidosis, ketosis (due to diabetes, starvation, or alcohol excess) and toxins (e.g. salicylates, methanol, propylene glycol, paraldehyde, ethylene glycol).

There is no standardized upper limit of normal for capillary ketones in pregnancy, but it is likely to be similar to that of non-pregnancy individuals (0.6 mmol/l). In this case, urinary and capillary ketones are increased. Urinary ketones (reflecting acetoacetate), whilst easy to perform, are inferior to capillary ketones (reflecting β-hydroxybutyrate) and the latter are preferred if ketoacidosis is suspected. The blood glucose is also low, which all lead to the most likely diagnosis being starvation ketoacidosis, related to vomiting and the period of reduced oral intake.

3. Why is this metabolic derangement more common in pregnancy?

Normally insulin suppresses ketone production by promoting glucose and carbohydrate metabolism over fat metabolism. However, in pregnancy, placental hormones lead to a state of insulin resistance, and there is also preferential transport of glucose and amino acids across the placenta to the fetus. Therefore in pregnancy, a relatively short period of reduced oral intake leads to increased fat metabolism, and with reduced insulin efficacy, ketogenesis can occur.

4. What is the likely underlying cause?

It is important to recognize that starvation ketoacidosis is the consequence rather than the cause of her initial symptoms and careful assessment for the underlying pathology should be undertaken in parallel to the treatment of the biochemical abnormalities.

In this case, the likely diagnosis is infection and bacterial tonsillitis, resulting in significantly reduced oral intake. Group A streptococcus infection is a cause of bacterial tonsillitis and is of particular concern in pregnancy (see Case 37). Appropriate antibiotics as guided by local antimicrobial guidelines should be prescribed.

Vomiting that starts after about 16 weeks of gestation cannot be attributed to pregnancy alone and assessment for the underlying cause should always be performed. Other causes of vomiting include pancreatitis, gastro-oesophageal reflux, and acute fatty liver of pregnancy.

5. What investigations would you arrange?

Arterial/venous blood gas is required as this enables assessment of the anion gap and is a way to monitor resolution of the metabolic derangement.

Regular assessment of ketosis using capillary ketones is required and should be repeated until readings normalize.

Capillary/serum glucose should be monitored regularly until the biochemical derangement recovers, as this may be affected by the treatment instituted for the ketosis.

Microbiological samples such as urine, stool, blood, and throat swabs should be taken and sent for culture, depending on the history, to confirm suspicions of an acute infective precipitant and to guide antibiotic choice and duration.

Chest radiography should be undertaken if there is any concern about a chest source of infection, or pathology that might be contributing to her tachypnoea. She is also at increased risk of aspiration given the history of vomiting. A low threshold for abdominal imaging would also be useful, typically with abdominal ultrasound to look for causes of vomiting such as gallstones, cholecystitis, or pancreatitis.

Fetal monitoring using continuous electronic fetal monitoring is likely to demonstrate a marked fetal tachycardia and may lead to an abnormal classification. It is very likely that this reflects maternal physiology and not fetal compromise so therefore immediate delivery is not always the best action.

6. How would you manage this woman?

Her care should be coordinated in an HDU or ITU setting, with a multidisciplinary approach, involving obstetricians, obstetric physicians, intensivists, neonatologists, and midwives.

Maternal

- Intravenous glucose provides both fuel for metabolism and can increase endogenous insulin production, leading to suppression of ketone production.
- A fixed rate intravenous insulin infusion can be given alongside glucose if the ketosis persists despite adequate glucose replacement and an increase in glucose level.
- Intravenous fluid replacement to treat dehydration and hypovolaemia.
- Regular monitoring of biochemical parameters including capillary ketones and glucose, venous pH and bicarbonate, renal function and serum sodium.
- Thiamine supplementation (oral or intravenous) should be considered if the vomiting has been more protracted.

- Antiemetics as needed.
- Do not give intravenous sodium bicarbonate for the correction of acidosis as this can worsen intracellular acidosis and lead to hypokalaemia and cerebral oedema.
- Evaluate the cause of the vomiting.
- Consider antibiotics according to local protocol if any suggestion of sepsis.

Fetal

- Regular fetal monitoring depending on gestational age.
- Delivery is determined by obstetric indications, for example if concerns about fetal monitoring despite maternal resuscitation. If the maternal condition is treated adequately as above, then delivery is rarely required.

Further reading

1. C. Frise *et al.* Starvation ketoacidosis in pregnancy. European Journal of Obstetrics, Gynaecology and Reproductive Biology. 2013; **167**: 1–7.

Case 15

A 30-year-old woman presented to her GP with a two-day history of dysuria, urinary frequency, and an offensive smell to her urine. She was 28 weeks into her first pregnancy. Her pregnancy had been uncomplicated apart from a previous urinary tract infection with similar symptoms 6 weeks prior to this presentation. A urine culture at that time had confirmed *E. coli*, sensitive to amoxicillin, so she was given a 5-day course, which led to resolution of her symptoms. She was otherwise fit and well with no past medical history, and was not taking any regular medications. She lived with her husband, worked as an accountant, and had never smoked.

Initial assessment

General inspection: Well in herself
Heart rate: 88 bpm
Blood pressure: 105/60 mmHg
Respiratory rate: 15 breaths/min
Temperature: 37.8 °C
Oxygen saturations: 99% on room air
Urinalysis: 1+ protein, 2+ leucocytes, 2+ blood, positive nitrites

Examination

Cardiovascular: Normal heart sounds, no murmurs
Respiratory: Normal breath sounds
Abdomen: Soft, mild suprapubic tenderness

Bloods

See Table 15.1.

Table 15.1 Bloods

Haemoglobin	111 g/L
WCC	14.2 × 10⁹/L
Platelets	188 × 10⁹/L
Sodium	138 mmol/L
Potassium	3.9 mmol/L
Urea	2.1 mmol/L
Creatinine	42 µmol/L
Bilirubin	7 µmol/L
ALT	12 iU/L
Albumin	29 g/L
CRP	56 mg/L

Questions

1. How useful is the urinalysis in this case?
2. Which investigations would you arrange for her?
3. Are you going to start treatment, and if so, what are the treatment options?
4. Are there any tests you would consider after this acute infection?
5. Would you start her on antibiotic prophylaxis after this infection is treated?

Answers

1. How useful is the urinalysis in this case?

Urine culture is the gold standard for the diagnosis of bacteriuria. Urinalysis are commonly performed in pregnancy looking for proteinuria but should not be relied upon as a confirmatory test for infection. The widespread use of strips that have multiple different reagents often generates information that was not the primary indication for doing the test.

Nitrites

A positive nitrite result suggests UTI (usually due to *E. coli*, *Klebsiella*, or *Proteus*), although some bacteria do not produce nitrites (e.g. *Staphylococcus*, *Streptococcus*, and *Haemophilus*) resulting in false negative nitrite testing.

Leucocytes

A positive result for leucocytes indicates pyuria, which in turn may constitute evidence of UTI, although this has a low positive predictive value in the absence of nitrites and symptoms, particularly in women. Contamination of a specimen with vaginal flora is a common cause of leucocyte positivity, limiting its diagnostic utility. It is not recommended that urine culture is performed in the presence of positive leucocytes alone.

Protein

There does not appear to be a clear correlation between the degree of proteinuria and the likelihood of urine infection, and urine infection is not a common cause of proteinuria. Therefore, it is difficult to advocate routine urine culture in the presence of protein only on the dipstick, although this is very commonly performed. New-onset proteinuria in pregnancy should always prompt review for pre-eclampsia.

Blood

False positives are common as urine may be contaminated by vaginal secretions or blood from haemorrhoids. However, recurrent dipstick haematuria (also known as 'microscopic' or 'non-visible') should prompt microscopic examination of urine for red cells as in many cases the dipstick positivity will not reflect the presence of red cells in the urine. This resolves after birth in most women but requires further investigation if it does not.

In this case, therefore, the findings on the urinalysis are supportive of the diagnosis of urinary tract infection, but ultimately the dipstick is not an essential part of the investigation for UTI. Treatment is indicated on symptoms alone, and urine culture is the gold standard for confirmation of infection.

2. Which investigations would you arrange for her?

Urine culture is the most important test to perform in anyone with symptoms suggestive of a UTI.

Significant growth (growth of a single organism at a level above 10^5 CFU/ml) may reflect both pathogenic and contaminant bacteria. If an unfamiliar organism is reported, it is advisable to check that this is not a probable contaminant before prescribing treatment.

Confusion often arises with other results reported on laboratory samples, which include:

Equivocal growth: the growth of a single organism, but only 10^4 to 10^5 CFU/ml so under the threshold deemed significant growth

Mixed growth: the growth of more than one organism on culture, with no single predominant organism, the most common cause of which is thought to be contamination of the urine sample.

Blood cultures are important if there is any suspicion of systemic infection.

A renal ultrasound is commonly considered, but in uncomplicated lower urinary tract infection is only required if there is a concern about structural conditions which might predispose to infection, suggested in the history, examination, or blood results. In upper urinary tract infection (i.e. pyelonephritis), a lower threshold for renal ultrasound should be used, as structural abnormalities are more common.

3. Are you going to start treatment, and if so, what are the treatment options?

The presence of urinary symptoms is enough to warrant empirical antibiotics, but if there is doubt that symptoms reflect urinary tract infection, it is appropriate to wait the short time until the urine culture result is available, and treatment started if bacteriuria identified.

Common antibiotics used to treat urinary infections include:

- **Cefalexin**
- **Amoxicillin** (avoid in penicillin allergy)
- **Nitrofurantoin** (first choice but avoid after 37 weeks of gestation or if birth is thought to be imminent, due to potential risk of neonatal haemolysis)
- **Trimethoprim** (avoid in the first trimester due to the risk of neural tube defects in the fetus; if given, supplement with folic acid 5 mg daily)

The order of preference depends on local antimicrobial policy which will reflect knowledge of local resistance patterns.

Less commonly antibiotics such as fosfomycin may be required, which can be used in pregnancy as normal. Gentamicin can be used in pregnancy, and a one-off dose for sepsis or a specific resistant organism is the most common regime encountered. Occasionally regular gentamicin is required, in which case levels should be monitored carefully. Amoxicillin and clavulanic acid use in pregnancy has been associated with an increased risk of necrotizing enterocolitis in babies born preterm, so this is often avoided if preterm birth is anticipated.

Antibiotics to avoid in pregnancy for treatment of UTI include ciprofloxacin. If in doubt with respect to choice of agent on grounds of allergy, drug interactions, resistant organisms, or contraindications, or if concerns about recurrent infection arise, then the case should be discussed with the Microbiology team.

4. Are there any tests you would consider after this acute infection?

If there is no bacterial growth on the initial urine culture, consideration should be given to alternative causes for the symptoms such as urethral syndrome, interstitial cystitis, painful bladder syndrome, or vulvovaginitis secondary to thrush, bacterial vaginosis, or sexually transmitted organisms.

In all women who receive a course of antibiotics for urine infection, urine culture should be repeated 7 days after finishing the treatment course. If the organism is still present, a further course of antibiotics to which the organism is sensitive should be prescribed.

5. Would you start her on antibiotic prophylaxis after this infection is treated?

Prophylactic antibiotics should only be considered in the context of recurrent infection with the same organism later in pregnancy after earlier confirmation of clearance of the infection following a complete treatment course of antibiotics. Opinions vary about the threshold for starting this; there is no clear agreement on whether two or three infections should prompt prophylaxis, but it is prudent to have a lower threshold in women with structural abnormalities, renal stones, or a kidney transplant.

Advice about adequate daily fluid intake, ensuring complete bladder emptying at each void, and vulval hygiene (such as voiding after sexual intercourse) is helpful in women with recurrent infection. It is also practical to provide a clean specimen container to these women so that a timely specimen can be collected if symptoms develop.

Further reading

1. NICE Clinical Knowledge Summary: Suspected urinary tract infection without visible haematuria during pregnancy. (last revised September 2022) <https://cks.nice.org.uk/topics/urinary-tract-infection-lower-women/management/uti-in-pregnancy-no-visible-haematuria/>.

Case 16

A 25-year-old woman attended her 16-week antenatal appointment with her midwife and mentioned she had developed intermittent pain affecting the small joints of both hands and wrists 10 months prior to this appointment, but they had become more problematic in the preceding 5 weeks. In addition, she had developed a facial rash, intermittent chest discomfort, and shortness of breath. This was her first pregnancy. Her booking BP was 117/70 mmHg and BMI was 27 kg/m². She took no medication, and she had no significant past medical history or family history. She did not smoke or drink alcohol. She was referred for urgent review.

Initial assessment

General inspection: Well; erythematous butterfly rash on face
Heart rate: 86 bpm
Blood pressure: 115/65 mmHg
Respiratory rate: 14 breaths/min
Temperature: 36.6 °C
Oxygen saturations: 99% on room air
Urinalysis: 1+ protein, 1+ blood

Examination

Cardiovascular: Normal heart sounds, no murmurs
Respiratory: Normal breath sounds
Abdomen: Soft abdomen, gravid uterus appropriate size for dates
Joints: Bilateral, symmetrical painful swelling of the proximal
                  interphalangeal joints, distal interphalangeal joints, and wrists

Bloods

See Table 16.1.

Table 16.1 Bloods

Haemoglobin	100 g/L
WCC	3.5×10^9/L
Platelets	110×10^9/L
Sodium	138 mmol/L
Potassium	4.1 mmol/L
Urea	2.3 mmol/L
Creatinine	48 µmol/L
Bilirubin	6 µmol/L
ALT	7 iU/L
ALP	70 iU/L
Albumin	34 g/L
CRP	7 mg/L
CK	125 U/L

Questions

1. What are the potential causes of her symptoms?
2. What other investigations would you like to perform?
3. How can you confirm the diagnosis?
4. She is found to be anti-Ro and La positive. How would you counsel her?
5. Investigations confirmed the likely diagnosis. What treatment would you start?

Answers

1. What are the potential causes of her symptoms?

Systemic lupus erythematosus (SLE) is suggested by the multisystem involvement with a malar rash, joint swelling, symptoms suggestive of pleuritis and pericarditis, as well as thrombocytopenia, leucopenia, and anaemia. SLE is a chronic multisystem autoimmune disorder of unknown aetiology, diagnosed in accordance with recently updated guidelines (see Figure 16.1).

Rheumatoid arthritis is a multisystem autoimmune disease, characterized by symmetrical painful swelling of small joints, often leading to characteristic deformities of the digits (swan neck, ulnar deviation) and erosive joint space destruction on plain radiographs. Extra-articular manifestations include serositis, fatigue, respiratory symptoms, and anaemia. Serological diagnosis is indicated by the presence of anti-cyclic citrullinated peptide (anti-CCP) antibodies. Rheumatoid factor can also be suggestive but is less specific than anti-CCP antibodies and can be positive in a variety of other autoimmune conditions.

Mixed connective tissue disease is characterized by overlapping features of SLE, systemic sclerosis, and polymyositis, and the presence of anti-RNP antibodies.

Undifferentiated connective tissue disease is suggested by signs and symptoms of multisystem autoimmune disease but which do not fit in to the classification criteria for any of the other autoimmune disease, nor the serological criteria.

Infections including CMV, EBV, and HIV can result in symptoms like those described here but are less likely due to the chronicity of the symptoms.

2. What other investigations would you like to perform?

Blood tests

Routine blood tests as above are required in all possible cases of inflammatory rheumatological disorders. Erythrocyte sedimentation rate (ESR), is elevated in pregnancy, so is less diagnostically useful in this scenario.

Urine

Urine microscopy should be sent to confirm the presence of red and/or white blood cells, as well as to establish whether casts are present. A urine protein:creatinine ratio should also be obtained.

Immunology

Anti-nuclear antibodies (ANA) are positive in almost all individuals with SLE, and if positive, should be further characterized by testing for extractable nuclear antigens (ENA).

Anti-double stranded DNA (dsDNA) antibodies are highly specific for SLE. Their titres can increase during a flare of disease, and this, combined with other manifestations of disease activity, can be useful in differentiating a flare of disease from other diagnoses.

Entry criterion
Antinuclear antibodies (ANA) at a titer of ≥ 1:80 on HEp-2 cells or an equivalent positive test (ever)

↓

If absent, do not classify as SLE If present, apply additive criteria

↓

Additive criteria
Do not count a criterion if there is a more likely explanation than SLE.
Occurrence of a criterion on at least one occasion is sufficient.
SLE classification requires at least one clinical criterion and ≥ 10 points.
Criteria need not occur simultaneously.
Within each domain, only the highest weighted criterion is counted toward the total score§.

Clinical domains and criteria	Weight	Immunology domains and criteria	Weight
Constitutional		*Antiphospholipid antibodies*	
Fever	2	Anti-cardiolipin antibodies OR	
Hematologic		Anti-β2GP1 antibodies OR	
Leucopenia	3	Lupus anticoagulant	2
Thrombocytopenia	4	*Complement proteins*	
Autoimmune haemolysis	4	Low C3 OR low C4	3
Neuropsychiatric		Low C3 AND low C4	4
Delirium	2	*SLE-specific antibodies*	
Psychosis	3	Anti-dsDNA antibody* OR	
Seizure	5	Anti-Smith antibody	6
Mucocutaneous			
Non-scarring alopecia	2		
Oral ulcers	2		
Subacute cutaneous OR discoid lupus	4		
Acute cutaneous lupus	6		
Serosal			
Pleural or pericardial effusion	5		
Acute pericarditis	6		
Musculoskeletal			
Joint involvement	6		
Renal			
Proteinuria > 0.5 g/24 h	4		
Renal biopsy Class II or V lupus nephritis	8		
Renal biopsy Class III or IV lupus nephritis	10		
Total score:			

↓

Classify as Systemic Lupus Erythematosus with a score of 10 or more if entry criterion fulfilled.

Figure 16.1 2019 European League against Rheumatism/American College of Rheumatology classification criteria for systemic lupus erythematosus. Reprinted from Aringer M *et al.* (2019). '2019 European League Against Rheumatism/American College of Rheumatology Classification Criteria for Systemic Lupus Erythematosus' *Arthritis and Rheumatology* with permission from John Wiley and Sons.

Complement C3 and C4 can fall in a lupus flare.

Anti-nuclear cytoplasmic antibody (ANCA) positivity points towards a vasculitic cause such as microscopic polyangiitis or granulomatosis with polyangiitis.

Anti-Ro/La antibodies are found to be positive in approximately 30% of individuals with SLE. They are relevant in pregnancy as these antibodies are associated with congenital heart block and neonatal cutaneous lupus.

Anti-RNP antibodies may be positive in mixed connective tissue disease.

Anti-Jo antibodies may be positive in patients with polymyositis and dermatomyositis.

Rheumatoid factor is non-specific and can be positive in a variety of autoimmune conditions.

Anti-CCP antibodies are more specific for rheumatoid arthritis.

Lupus anticoagulant/anti-cardiolipin antibodies are suggestive of a diagnosis of antiphospholipid syndrome, which can occur in individuals with SLE (known as secondary antiphospholipid syndrome). However these fluctuate rapidly, so must be positive on two samples taken 12 weeks or more apart to be diagnostically significant.

Serology

HIV should have been performed as part of the antenatal screening bloods but needs to be performed at this point if it was not done earlier in pregnancy, or there is uncertainty about the results.

Viral serology for EBV, CMV, hepatitis B, and parvovirus B19 is advised if the symptoms of arthralgia have been present for less than 6 weeks.

Other investigations

Echocardiography should be considered to evaluate her symptoms of shortness of breath and chest discomfort, in order to look for evidence of myopericarditis or any valvular abnormalities.

Chest radiography should be performed, given her shortness of breath and chest discomfort. Cross-sectional imaging is required if there is a concern about pulmonary embolism.

Joint imaging can be considered, for example ultrasound looking for effusion or plain radiography looking for joint erosion.

3. What is required to confirm the diagnosis?

There are a variety of diagnostic criteria that exist for the diagnosis of SLE, including the American College of Rheumatology (ACR, 2012) and the European League against Rheumatism (EULAR, 2019) diagnostic criteria.

4. She is found to be anti-Ro and La positive. How would you counsel her?

These antibodies, whilst markers of underlying autoimmune conditions, do not have any clinical effects in non-pregnant individuals. However they can cross the placenta and cause congenital heart block. This occurs in approximately 2% of antibody-positive women, but if one pregnancy is affected, there is a much higher chance of the next pregnancy being affected (17–20% in studies). The presence of anti-Ro/La antibodies therefore should prompt specialist fetal echocardiography, as well as regular fetal heart auscultation from 16–20 weeks of gestation onwards.

There is evidence that hydroxychloroquine in women with a previously affected pregnancy reduces the recurrence risk from 17–20% to about 7%. There is no evidence yet to support hydroxychloroquine use in all women with anti-Ro/La antibodies without a previously affected pregnancy, but some centres advocate this approach.

These antibodies are also associated with a 5% risk of neonatal cutaneous lupus, which is a transient, florid, non-scarring, reticulate rash. The rash resolves as the neonate clears the antibodies. Sometimes the antibody status of the mother is not recognized as a potential cause of the neonatal rash, so some babies undergo investigations which are ultimately not required.

5. Investigations confirmed the likely diagnosis. What treatment would you start?

During pregnancy this woman should be under joint care with Rheumatology.

Acute treatment with glucocorticoids is typically used initially, as well as a treatment for flares of the disease in pregnancy. The dose can be tapered as her symptoms settle.

Optimisation of treatment with medications including hydroxychloroquine, sulfa-salazine, and azathioprine can be achieved in pregnancy.

Fetal monitoring with serial growth scans in the late second and third trimesters is recommended due to the increased risk of fetal growth restriction in association with a flare of SLE.

Monitoring for pre-eclampsia is required, as active SLE is associated with an increased risk. Low-dose aspirin, started prior to 16 weeks of gestation and continued until the late third trimester, is safe to take and is proven to improve pregnancy outcomes in women at risk of pre-eclampsia.

VTE prophylaxis with LMWH would usually be recommended in active lupus unless contra-indications are present. Thrombocytopenia below a level of 50×10^9/L warrants discussion with a Haematologist. If there is impaired renal function, then reduced doses should be used.

The patient responded well to the steroids and her symptoms settled. At 28 weeks of gestation she was readmitted with a worsening of her rash, new hypertension, and proteinuria. Her blood results showed an increase in creatinine and thrombocytopenia.

Question

6. What might help distinguish pre-eclampsia from a lupus flare?

Answer

6. What might help distinguish pre-eclampsia from a lupus flare?

It can be difficult to differentiate a flare of SLE from evolving pre-eclampsia as both can present with similar features including hypertension, proteinuria, thrombocytopenia, and deteriorating renal function. There are, however, more specific blood markers that can help in the diagnosis. A fall in complement (C3 and C4), and an increase in dsDNA titre are suggestive of a flare of SLE. The newly available serum biomarkers placental growth factor (PLGF) and soluble fms-like tyrosine kinase 1 (sFlt-1) levels can be used to stratify risk of imminent pre-eclampsia; a low PLGF level or a high sFlt-1/PLGF ratio is suggestive of higher risk.

Further reading

1. M. Knight and C. Nelson-Piercy. Management of SLE during pregnancy: challenges and solutions. Open Access Rheumatology. 2017; 9: 37–53.
2. EULAR recommendations for the management of systemic lupus erythematosus (2019 update). 2019. <https://www.eular.org/myUploadData/files/eular_recommendation_sle_press_release_4_april_2019.pdf>

Case 17

A 32-year-old woman presented to the Emergency Department at 26 weeks of gestation with a vague constellation of worsening symptoms. She had a 4-week history of intractable nausea and was unable to tolerate oral fluids, despite treatment with cyclizine, metoclopramide, and ondansetron. She had also been experiencing intermittent generalized abdominal cramps, associated with loose stool, which was occasionally streaked with blood. She had been feeling increasingly tired, light-headed, and short of breath on minimal exertion. This was her first pregnancy, and she had no past medical history. In addition to the antiemetics, she was taking ferrous sulphate 200 mg on alternate days, as anaemia was identified on her booking bloods. Her father had a history of colonic polyps. She was an ex-smoker (10–15 a day for 12 years) and had drunk 25 units of alcohol per week prior to pregnancy. There was no history of recent overseas travel.

Initial assessment

General inspection:	Evidence of weight loss and reduced muscle mass, particularly around shoulders
	Dehydrated
Heart rate:	118 bpm
Blood pressure:	90/60 mmHg
Respiratory rate:	20 breaths/min
Temperature:	37.8 °C
Oxygen saturations:	95% on room air
Urinalysis:	1+ protein

Examination

Cardiovascular:	Normal heart sounds, no murmurs
Respiratory:	Normal breath sounds
Abdomen:	Soft distended abdomen; difficult to palpate uterus clearly, suspicion of ascites
Lymph nodes:	No cervical, axillary, or inguinal lymphadenopathy
Breasts:	No lumps

Bloods

See Table 17.1.

Table 17.1 Bloods

Haemoglobin	90 g/L
WCC	13×10^9/L
Platelets	550×10^9/L
Sodium	135 mmol/L
Potassium	4.1 mmol/L
Urea	2.9 mmol/L
Creatinine	45 µmol/L
Bilirubin	35 µmol/L
ALT	200 iU/L
ALP	500 iU/L
Albumin	25 g/L
CRP	40 mg/L
Amylase	50 U/L
Glucose	6.1 mmol/L
Bile acids	6 µmol/l

Questions

1. What initial tests are required, in addition to those already performed?
2. What are the potential causes of her symptoms?
3. What other investigations would you like to perform?

Answers

1. What initial tests are required, in addition to those already performed?

More specific *blood tests* are warranted, given the abnormalities on the initial bloods. These include blood film, ferritin, B12, and folate, screen for liver autoantibodies and hepatitis serology (A, B, C, and E), calcium, and blood cultures.

Microbiological samples including urine and stool samples are also important to perform.

Faecal calprotectin is a helpful marker of bowel inflammation.

Chest radiograph is important to look for specific causes of breathlessness.

Abdominal ultrasound would be advisable given the abnormal liver function tests.

2. What are the potential causes of her symptoms?

Inflammatory bowel disease (IBD) includes ulcerative colitis and Crohn's disease and is common in this age group. Presenting symptoms include bloody diarrhoea, abdominal pain, change in bowel habit, and mucus in the stool. Endoscopy can be performed in pregnancy if required.

Infection should always be considered in those with symptoms of abdominal pain and loose stool. If there is associated bloody diarrhoea, bacteria such as *E. coli*, *Shigella*, and *Campylobacter* are common causes, but these are less likely here due to the duration of her symptoms. Infective organisms such as *C. difficile* and *Giardia* should be considered, as these can often produce longer lasting symptoms, however, the latter is less likely in the context of bloody stools.. *C. difficile* is often associated with preceding antibiotic use.

Malignancy, in particular metastatic solid organ malignancy, is a potential cause of these symptoms. Common malignancies presenting in pregnancy include breast cancer, colorectal cancer, ovarian cancer, melanoma, and cervical cancer, however many malignancies may present at an advanced stage in pregnancy.

Pancreatitis should be considered in all patients with abdominal pain and abnormal LFTs. Pancreatitis can be acute or chronic and is often related to the presence of gallstones. Whilst an increased amylase is a useful indicator of acute pancreatitis, this is often normal in chronic pancreatitis.

Coeliac disease is an autoimmune condition associated with duodenal villous atrophy and crypt hyperplasia, and symptoms related to gluten intolerance. It often occurs in conjunction with other autoimmune conditions, such as type 1 diabetes and hypothyroidism. Symptoms include steatorrhoea and abdominal pain in relation to food containing gluten. This is unlikely in this woman as she has bloody stools (which are not a feature of coeliac disease), other symptoms that cannot be attributed to coeliac disease, no obvious food triggers, and no history of autoimmune disease.

3. What other investigations would you like to perform?

Cross-sectional imaging is urgently required, and a common combination in pregnancy is to perform CT imaging of chest ± neck if required, and MRI of the abdomen +/− pelvis. Iodinated contrast for CT imaging can be used as normal in pregnancy. Gadolinium for MRI is discouraged, but this can be used in certain circumstances where no alternative is possible and this is essential for diagnosis (e.g. to aid characterization of liver lesions).

Biopsy is the key test for individuals with metastatic disease and the best location for this is usually identified on cross-sectional imaging. This may be of a metastatic deposit (but a liver biopsy would ideally be avoided in pregnancy) or an accessible lymph node. Often a potential primary lesion is identified on imaging, for example a colonic lesion, so direct visualization with endoscopy can be performed which would also facilitate tissue biopsies. Colonoscopy and gastroscopy under sedation can be performed at any gestation of pregnancy, provided practical attention is paid to patient positioning.

She was given IV fluid, antiemetics and analgesia. Blood testing showed increased calcium (2.95 mmol/L), and the liver screen did not identify any abnormalities. The abdominal ultrasound showed multiple lesions in the liver in all lobes, consistent with metastatic disease.

CTPA showed no pulmonary emboli and no evidence of primary or secondary malignancy. An MRI abdomen confirmed large volume liver metastases, and a lesion in the transverse colon causing significant narrowing of the lumen, consistent with a primary colorectal cancer. A colonoscopy was performed, where biopsies of the transverse colon lesion were taken. These confirmed adenocarcinoma. Treatment options including chemotherapy (oxaliplatin, 5-FU, and folinic acid) were discussed.

Question

4. How would you treat her?

Answer

4. How would you treat her?

Treatment of anaemia

Replacement of iron, B12, or folate should be undertaken if identified (bearing in mind the normal range for B12 is lower in pregnancy so results should be interpreted carefully). Blood transfusion may be required if no deficiency is identified to optimize her haemoglobin prior to chemotherapy.

Treatment of her malignancy

Many chemotherapeutic agents have been used successfully in pregnancy. Use is generally avoided in the first trimester and should be stopped 2–3 weeks prior to the anticipated delivery date, to minimize the chances of neutropenia at the time of birth. Oxaliplatin and fluorouracil have been used in pregnancy, however there is limited evidence regarding the use of capecitabine. The use of these chemotherapy agents is therefore appropriate in this case.

Surgical intervention can be performed in pregnancy if required, for example if she developed bowel obstruction from the tumour. The timing and practicalities of surgery depend on gestational age and require multidisciplinary discussion.

Fetal monitoring

Chemotherapy can be associated with growth restriction, so serial growth scans are usually advised.

Birth plans

The diagnosis of malignancy is not necessarily an indication for preterm birth, unless specific fetal concerns arise, or the mother becomes unwell for example with sepsis. However early delivery may be planned in some cases, balancing the competing risks of delayed resection of the tumour versus preterm birth.

VTE prophylaxis

This is required in all women with active malignancy, unless specific contraindications exist (e.g. low platelets) when mechanical thromboprophylaxis should be advised as an alternative.

Further reading

1. **J. Rogers** *et al.* Colorectal cancer during pregnancy or postpartum: case series and literature review. Obstetric Medicine. 2022: 15; 118–124. <https://doi.org/10.1177/1753495X211041228>

Case 18

A 35-year-old woman with type 1 diabetes mellitus was pregnant for the first time. Her glycaemic control prior to conception was very good (pre-conception HbA1c 42 mmol/mol) and she had no history of retinopathy or nephropathy. She had an insulin pump and used continuous glucose monitoring. At booking her BP was 105/65 mmHg and BMI was 21 kg/m². She also had a history of vitiligo. She was taking folic acid 5 mg daily, vitamin D 1000 units daily, and aspirin 150 mg daily. Her family history was notable for rheumatoid arthritis and hypothyroidism in her mother. She did not smoke or drink alcohol.

She attended the specialist diabetes clinic at 28 weeks and no changes were made to her pump settings. She reported some nausea and intermittent, mild abdominal pain so was asked to attend the Maternity Assessment Unit where she was assessed, and blood tests were sent.

Initial assessment

General inspection: Well
Heart rate: 90 bpm
Blood pressure: 110/70 mmHg
Respiratory rate: 12 breaths/min
Temperature: 36.4 °C
Oxygen saturations: 99% on room air
Urinalysis: No protein

Examination

Cardiovascular: Normal heart sounds, no murmurs
Respiratory: Normal breath sounds
Abdomen: Soft abdomen; gravid uterus appropriate size for dates
Cervix: Os closed, no sign of rupture of membranes

Bloods

See Table 18.1.

Table 18.1 Bloods

Haemoglobin	110 g/L
WCC	6.5 × 10⁹/L
Platelets	100 × 10⁹/L
Sodium	135 mmol/L
Potassium	3.9 mmol/L
Urea	2.3 mmol/L
Creatinine	44 µmol/L
Bilirubin	20 µmol/L
ALT	900 iU/L
ALP	200 iU/L
Albumin	28 g/L
CRP	15 mg/L
PT	12 s
APTT	24 s

Questions

1. What abnormalities of liver function tests are shown here?
2. What are the possible causes of her abnormal liver function tests?
3. Which additional investigations would you like to perform?

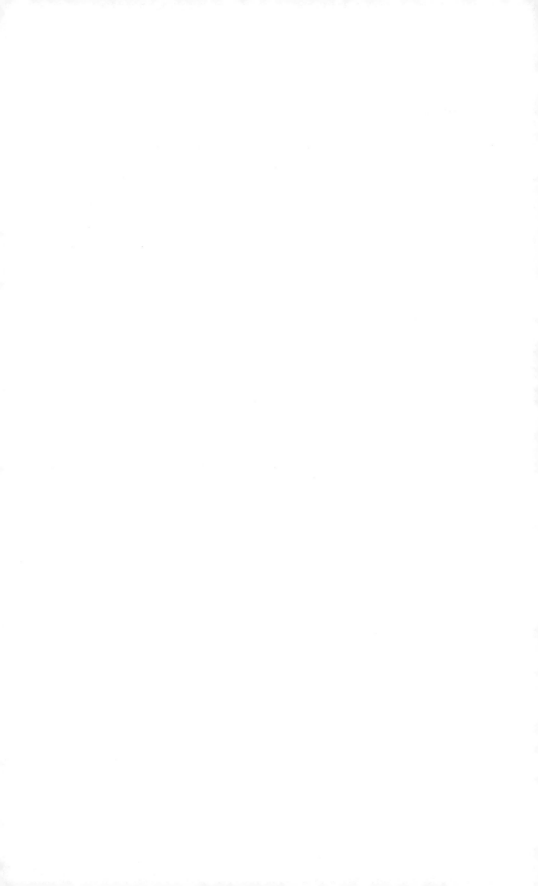

Answers

1. What abnormalities of liver function tests are shown here?

The results show a rise in transaminases to a greater degree than the rise in alkaline phosphatase. Alkaline phosphatase often increases in pregnancy due to production of the placental isoenzyme, up to about three times the upper limit of normal, but in a subgroup of women much higher levels are seen. This increase in transaminases is significant and concerning, however is not associated with impaired synthetic function at this time (no changes in glucose control, normal coagulation parameters, and normal albumin).

2. What are the possible causes of her abnormal liver function tests?

Viruses (particularly hepatitis A and E, CMV, EBV, HSV) can cause acute increases in transaminases so a thorough travel, dietary, drug, and sexual history is important.

Medications commonly affect liver function, and so a careful medication history is important, including prescribed, over-the-counter, and recreational drugs. Medications used in pregnancy that can cause a rise in transaminases include omeprazole, SSRIs, and rifampicin. Other medications include paracetamol and herbal or Chinese medications.

Autoimmune hepatitis can cause elevated transaminases. The patient described here has a personal and family history of autoimmune conditions which increase the likelihood of another autoimmune condition arising.

Intrahepatic cholestasis of pregnancy (ICP) is defined as pruritus in association with raised bile acids, in the absence of any other cause. There can also be an associated transaminitis. It is a diagnosis of exclusion, however, so all other causes must be considered.

Non-alcoholic fatty liver disease (NAFLD) is a common cause of abnormal LFTs and it reflects excess accumulation of triglycerides in the absence of significant alcohol intake, drugs, and viruses. It may present only with asymptomatic elevation of transaminases and is likely to be under-recognized in pregnancy. It can occur with insulin resistance and frequently occurs in individuals with metabolic syndrome, which is not the phenotype described in this patient.

Other causes include malignancy of any type affecting the liver (primary or secondary), systemic causes such as sepsis and heart failure and hereditary conditions such as α1-antitrypsin deficiency, hereditary haemochromatosis, and Wilson's disease.

3. What additional investigations would you like to perform?

Bloods including bile acids, viral serology (hepatitis A, hepatitis B surface antigen, hepatitis C antibody, hepatitis E IgM, EBV, CMV, and HIV), autoantibodies (antinuclear antibodies, anti-smooth muscle antibodies, anti-liver-kidney-microsome-1

(LKM1) antibodies, anti-liver cytosol antibodies, anti-mitochondrial antibodies), and immunoglobulins are advised.

Imaging is important to check for structural causes of these abnormalities, and ultrasound is an easy and accessible first-line investigation. MRI or MRCP can be considered if indicated by bloods or ultrasound findings. Transient elastography is used outside of pregnancy to evaluate liver cirrhosis, however this is not useful in pregnancy as liver stiffness increases.

Liver biopsy is rarely indicated in pregnancy, and there is concern about an increased bleeding risk, so this should only be performed if the result would change management in pregnancy and no alternative diagnostic test was an option.

Additional blood tests show that she has a high ANA titre (1 in 320), hypergammaglobulinaemia, and is positive for anti-smooth muscle antibodies.

4. How would you treat her?

The diagnosis of autoimmune hepatitis is suspected, so she requires discussion with Hepatology colleagues and consideration of treatment with steroids. Other immunosuppressants including ciclosporin and tacrolimus are also options in pregnancy. Azathioprine can also be used for maintenance of remission in pregnancy, but mycophenolate mofetil should be avoided. Steroid use will lead to a worsening of her glycaemic control, so liaison with her specialist diabetes team as well as patient education about insulin dose adjustments would be essential if steroids were started.

Her liver function should be assessed regularly, as should her bile acids in case superimposed cholestasis develops.

The aim for treatment is to optimize medical management irrespective of pregnancy status. The diagnosis is not an indication for delivery, but delivery decisions later in pregnancy should be individualized. It is likely that in this case the delivery timing will be determined by the type 1 diabetes rather than her liver condition.

4. How would you treat her?

Case 19

A 33-year-old woman was referred for pre-conception counselling because of cystic fibrosis. The diagnosis was made after she developed meconium ileus as a neonate, requiring surgical intervention at 3 days of age. She had continued to experience constipation into adulthood, requiring intermittent use of gastrograffin. Her weight was stable (BMI 21 kg/m²). She had experienced a great improvement in her condition since she started a combination CFTR protein modulator treatment. The latest forced expiratory volume (FEV1) was 62%.

Her medications included triple combination therapy (tezacaftor, ivacaftor, elexacaftor), DNAse nebulizer, salbutamol inhaler, tiotropium inhaler, colomycin nebulizer, steroid nasal spray, steroid inhaler, azithromycin, pancrealipase capsules, multivitamins, folic acid, macrogol, and omeprazole.

Questions

1. How does cystic fibrosis affect fertility?
2. What features are associated with adverse pregnancy outcomes?
3. How does pregnancy affect cystic fibrosis symptoms?
4. What specific screening does this woman require in pregnancy?
5. What would you advise regarding her medication in pregnancy?
6. What other advice should this woman receive to ensure she has an optimal pregnancy experience and outcome?

Answers

1. How does cystic fibrosis affect fertility?

Cystic fibrosis (CF) is associated with subfertility because of both the impact of mal-nutrition and chronic illness on the hypothalamic control of ovulation as well as the barrier effect of increased viscosity of the cervical mucus. However, new therapies such as triple combination therapy are transforming the course of the condition and are contributing to an improvement in fertility. All women who do not wish to be-come pregnant should be counselled about the contraception. Cystic fibrosis is not a contraindication to any form of contraception.

Men with CF are often infertile due to congenital absence of the vas deferens.

2. What features are associated with adverse pregnancy outcomes?

Reduced FEV1 (less than 50%) is associated with increased risk of caesarean de-livery, lower birth weight, and preterm birth. Lung function often declines in preg-nancy, but the degree of decline is not related to baseline lung function.

Women with cystic fibrosis have an increased risk of having infants with con-genital abnormalities (up to 2.5 times the background population risk) but no spe-cific risk factors for this have been identified.

Burkholderia cepacia colonization is a poor prognostic marker in all individuals with CF and is associated with an increased risk of death in pregnancy.

3. How does pregnancy affect cystic fibrosis symptoms?

With advancing pregnancy, the gravid uterus displaces the diaphragm and can im-pair sputum expectoration, which may worsen lung symptoms in pregnancy. There is an increased risk of pulmonary exacerbations requiring hospitalization and intra-venous antibiotics compared to when women are not pregnant, however these data were collected from populations prior to widespread use of CTFR receptor modulators.

The slowing of gastrointestinal motility seen in pregnancy can result in worsening of the typical gastrointestinal symptoms of cystic fibrosis, particularly in women who have suffered from distal intestinal obstruction syndrome.

Increased oestrogen production in pregnancy causes tissue oedema that can lead to increased nasal congestion, snoring, and obstructive sleep apnoea.

4. What additional screening does this woman require in pregnancy?

Due to the high risk of cystic fibrosis-related diabetes (CFRD), women with cystic fibrosis should undergo screening for diabetes early in the second trimester, and if normal, this should be repeated at 24–28 weeks of gestation. A 2-hour 75 g oral glucose tolerance test can be used, with the same criteria for a diagnosis of gestational diabetes, though capillary blood glucose monitoring may also be acceptable to establish the diagnosis.

Women with cystic fibrosis often gain less weight in pregnancy than those without CF so they therefore require regular monitoring and appropriate dietetic input to ensure adequate nutritional intake and weight gain. Fat-soluble vitamin levels should be checked every trimester and supplemented as appropriate.

With respect to inheritance, the partners of women with cystic fibrosis should be offered screening for heterozygosity for the *CFTR* gene mutation. If the woman's partner is a carrier, then the couple have a 50% risk of having a baby affected by CF. In this scenario, pre-implantation genetic diagnosis following IVF offers couples the chance to select only unaffected embryos for pregnancy. If a couple chooses not to pursue this option, or the carrier status of the partner is unknown, then prenatal diagnosis by invasive techniques (amniocentesis or chorionic villus sampling) is offered although these methods carry a risk of miscarriage (1% and 2% respectively). Developments in non-invasive prenatal diagnostic techniques (analysis of cell-free fetal DNA circulating in maternal serum) have increased the range of diseases that can be detected, and some laboratories offer testing for CF with this method. If the fetus is diagnosed with CF, then the parents can be sensitively counselled and offered a choice of continuing the pregnancy or choosing a termination.

5. What would you advise regarding her medication in pregnancy?

As with women with any chronic disease, women with cystic fibrosis must be counselled that the risks of any medication must be balanced against the risk of destabilizing their condition.

Though there are limited data on CFTR receptor modulators in pregnancy, they do not appear to be associated with adverse pregnancy outcomes. Women should be supported to continue them in pregnancy to maintain optimal lung function. However, as rodent studies suggest these drugs can cause cataracts, it is suggested that infants and children exposed to CFTR receptor modulators *in utero* undergo regular ophthalmic screening.

The use of DNAase nebulizers is not associated with adverse pregnancy outcomes and can be continued throughout pregnancy, as can the other inhalers (salbutamol, steroids and tiotropium) and steroid nasal spray.

Azithromycin and other macrolides are safe in pregnancy, as is nebulized colomycin to treat *Pseudomonas* colonization. If additional antibiotics are required to treat infection during pregnancy, it is advisable that this is done in conjunction with specialist Microbiology advice as well as the obstetric team.

Pancrealipase capsules should be continued through pregnancy. Cystic fibrosis-specific multivitamins should also be continued but should be reviewed for content and type of vitamin A since some vitamin A is teratogenic in excess.

Regular laxatives are important to avoid cystic fibrosis and pregnancy-related constipation.

6. What other advise should this woman receive to ensure she has an optimal pregnancy experience and outcome?

Folic acid is important for all pregnant women, from 3 months prior to conception to at least 12 weeks of gestation. A higher dose will be required if the woman has CFRD.

Women should be encouraged to continue with regular effective airway clearance and nebulizers to prevent a pulmonary exacerbation. Postural drainage techniques are not contra-indicated provided the uterus is accounted for and body positioning is supported appropriately. Oscillating positive expiratory pressure devices are safe to use. Physiotherapists should be part of the multidisciplinary team to assist with airway clearance, as well as the provision of advice on maintaining physical activity during pregnancy and pelvic floor exercises. Support for good cystic fibrosis self-management is particularly important after birth, where women often have a decline in lung function as they are less able to undertake lung clearance and continue with their optimal medication schedule while looking after a new baby.

Further reading

1. **M. Shteinberg** *et al.* Fertility and pregnancy in cystic fibrosis. Chest. 2021; **160** (6): 2051–60.
2. **Q. Reynaud** *et al.* Pregnancy outcome in women with cystic fibrosis and poor pulmonary function; Journal of Cystic Fibrosis. 2020; **19**(1): 80–3.
3. **A. Moran** *et al.* Clinical care guidelines for cystic fibrosis-related diabetes. A position statement of the American Diabetes Association and a clinical practice guideline of the Cystic Fibrosis Foundation, endorsed by the Pediatric Endocrine Society. Diabetes Care. 2010; 33(12): 2697–708.

Case 20

A 37-year-old woman was pregnant for the first time, with DCDA twins. She had an uncomplicated pregnancy and elective caesarean delivery was undertaken at 37 weeks of gestation. The twins were born in good condition with normal birthweight. Birth was complicated by postpartum haemorrhage; the mother lost approximately 400 ml of blood. She had no significant past medical history and her only regular medication in pregnancy was vitamin D and aspirin 150 mg daily (pre-eclampsia prophylaxis).

Immediately postpartum she had a single episode of hypertension (150/95 mmHg) that was normal when repeated. The day after birth it was noted that her urine output reduced significantly. The day after this, she complained of feeling generally unwell, with blurred vision and dizziness. She did not have a headache and had no altered level of consciousness.

Initial assessment

General inspection: GCS 15, bruising on upper limbs with scattered petechiae
                       Pitting oedema to mid-calf
Heart rate: 92 bpm
Blood pressure: 138/84 mmHg
Respiratory rate: 14 breaths/min
Temperature: 36.1 °C
Oxygen saturations: 98% on room air
Urinalysis: 1+ protein, 1+ blood

Examination

Cardiovascular: Normal heart sounds, no murmurs
Respiratory: Normal breath sounds
Abdomen: Well-contracted uterus; clean caesarean section wound
Arms: Bruising with scattered petechiae
Legs: Pitting oedema to mid-calf

Bloods

See Table 20.1.

Table 20.1 Bloods

	2 days before birth	Day 2 post-birth
Haemoglobin	121 g/l	76 g/l
WCC	6.3×10^9/l	10.1×10^9/l
Platelets	105×10^9/l	45×10^9/l
Sodium	138 mmol/l	142 mmol/l
Potassium	3.9 mmol/l	4.9 mmol/l
Urea	2.3 mmol/l	8 mmol/l
Creatinine	75 µmol/l	318 µmol/l
ALT	30 iU/L	25 iU/L
Urine PCR	Not done	956 mg/mmol

Questions

1. What are the possible diagnoses?
2. What other tests would you undertake?
3. How do you treat her?

Answers

1. What are the possible diagnoses?

The constellation of abnormalities shown here suggest a thrombotic microangiopathy (TMA). This range of conditions is suggested by anaemia, thrombocytopenia, renal damage, and neurological symptoms. The severity of these abnormalities, however, means that careful consideration should be given to other conditions that can cause a similar clinical picture and a thorough history, examination, and investigation is required to clarify the diagnosis. Some TMAs require supportive treatment alone, while some require targeted treatment to increase the chance of a good recovery.

Atypical haemolytic uraemic syndrome (HUS) is characterized by a triad of microangiopathic haemolytic anaemia, thrombocytopenia, and acute kidney injury. Other symptoms include headache, confusion, seizures, and abdominal pain. Severe renal dysfunction is typical, and therefore HUS is the most likely cause of symptoms in this case. The majority of people with HUS require dialysis at least temporarily, and many develop chronic kidney disease requiring long-term renal replacement therapy. Significant haemolysis is also very common in atypical HUS.

In pregnancy, atypical HUS is rare, but more common than typical HUS (often associated with gastroenteritis-related organisms such as *E. coli* and characterized by diarrhoea).

Thrombotic thrombocytopenic purpura (TTP) is a rare TMA. Historically, TTP was associated with a pentad of thrombocytopenia, haemolytic anaemia, acute kidney injury, fever, and altered mental status, though it is now widely recognized that not all features are needed for a diagnosis to be made or treatment to be started. TTP is associated with a deficiency in the enzyme ADAMTS13, usually due to acquired inhibitory autoantibodies, but occasionally from inherited mutations in the *ADAMTS13* gene. ADAMTS13 cleaves von Willebrand factor, so deficiency results in ultra-large multimers of VWF accumulating on the endothelial wall, and subsequent accumulation and attachment of platelets, leading to thrombocytopenia and MAHA.

The diagnosis is made by identifying a severe reduction in ADAMTS13 level. It should be noted that levels of this protease decrease in the third trimester of pregnancy, but not to a clinically significant degree. Specialist input is required if TTP is identified as affected individuals require rapid treatment.

It is important to consider this diagnosis in any woman where the clinical picture does not clearly fit with a hypertensive disorder of pregnancy, as delays in the diagnosis lead to an increased associated mortality. A low threshold for sending a blood sample for ADAMTS13 level is therefore advised.

The syndrome of haemolysis, elevated liver enzymes, and low platelets (HELLP) is the most common TMA in pregnancy. It typically occurs in women with pre-eclampsia, but importantly 20% occur without hypertension or proteinuria. Women with HELLP may have malaise, nausea, and vomiting, and may experience hypochondrial or epigastric pain. HELLP typically resolves 48–72 hours after birth. HELLP is less likely in this case as the transaminases are normal and the renal dysfunction and anaemia are severe.

Severe pre-eclampsia is characterized by hypertension, renal dysfunction, thrombocytopenia, elevated liver enzymes, neurological disturbance, and pulmonary oedema. Though pre-eclampsia is common, pre-eclampsia with severe features is less common.

In addition to TMAs, *haemorrhage* (i.e. significant acute blood loss) can cause anaemia and acute renal failure. Thrombocytopenia, however, is less likely in acute haemorrhage. It is very plausible that the clinical picture described above could develop in women with accumulating pathologies, for example, pre-eclampsia and postpartum haemorrhage or NSAID use (often given routinely after caesarean delivery).

Distinguishing the different conditions can be difficult, and discussion in a multidisciplinary team with experts in TMAs in pregnancy can help ensure the correct diagnosis is made.

2. What other tests would you undertake?

Urgent haematology samples for FBC and blood film are required, as well as reticulocytes and haptoglobin, which if abnormal would be consistent with haemolysis. LDH is a marker of haemolysis and can be very high in women with aHUS but is not specific to this condition and is moderately elevated in other TMAs. A direct antiglobulin test will exclude immune-mediated causes.

An ADAMTS13 level is required urgently, as if this is low, TTP is likely, which can be life-threatening if untreated and needs urgent intervention.

A renal ultrasound would also be useful to see if there are any structural abnormalities contributing to the renal impairment. If intra-operative ureteric injury is suspected (this may occur following surgical control of broad ligament or pelvic sidewall bleeding) then a CT ureterogram should be requested.

3. How do you treat her?

The abnormalities in this case are more suggestive of aHUS or TTP, rather than severe pre-eclampsia or HELLP. After ADAMTS13 activity has been tested and is normal (this excludes TTP), and a microangiopathic appearance on the blood film has been identified, it is important to start treatment for aHUS. Eculizumab, a monoclonal antibody that inhibits terminal complement activation at the C5 protein, is a specific treatment for HUS.

Careful fluid replacement is important, to ensure that the woman remains euvolaemic. Renal replacement therapy such as haemodialysis may be needed depending on the severity of the renal dysfunction. Platelet and red blood cell transfusions are given to support women if symptomatic or if they require an invasive procedure.

Plasma exchange is an effective treatment for TTP, but there is less evidence of benefit in other TMA syndromes including aHUS. If there is diagnostic uncertainty or delay in ADAMTS13 testing then women with aHUS may require a trial of plasma exchange, but this should be stopped as soon as the diagnosis of aHUS is made. Plasma exchange for TTP is usually used alongside other therapies, such as high-dose steroids or biologic agents (e.g. rituximab). Occasionally platelet transfusion and/or red cell transfusion are administered, for example in the setting of severe bleeding or if procedures are planned, but their use should be discussed with Haematology.

The mechanism of action of eculizumab results in the recipient being at increased risk of infection with *Meningococcus sp*. It is therefore important to ensure meningococcal vaccination is offered at an early stage, but also that the patient and healthcare professionals involved in their care are aware of this increased risk and understand the need to seek medical attention early if symptoms arise.

Further reading

1. **M. Gupta** *et al*. Thrombotic microangiopathies of pregnancy: Differential Diagnosis. Pregnancy Hypertension. 2018; **12**: 29–34.
2. BMJ Best Practice Haemolytic Uraemic Syndrome, October 2019 (reviewed October 2021) <https://bestpractice.bmj.com/topics/en-gb/470>

Case 21

A 35-year-old woman in her first pregnancy was referred to the maternal assessment unit at 36 weeks of gestation. During a routine midwifery appointment, her left eye had been noted to be red. She had noticed a gritty and irritated sensation. This had started 24 hours previously, and was not associated with any discharge, pain, or visual disturbance. There was no photophobia and no history or sensation suggestive of a foreign body. There was no history of injury, and she did not wear contact lenses.

She was known to have Crohn's disease and enteropathic arthritis. Prior to pregnancy she was treated with methotrexate and infliximab, but she had stopped all medications at conception. She was taking no medications except pregnancy multivitamins. A mild flare of arthritis earlier in the pregnancy had been treated with prednisolone. The pregnancy had otherwise been uneventful. She did not smoke or drink alcohol.

Initial assessment

General inspection: GCS 15/15. No cervical lymphadenopathy.
Heart rate: 80 bpm, regular
Blood pressure: 115/55 mmHg
Respiratory rate: 14 breaths/minute
Oxygen saturations: 98% on room air
Temperature: 36.9 °C
Urinalysis: No protein

Examination

Cardiovascular: Normal heart sounds, no added sounds
Respiratory: Normal breath sounds throughout
Abdomen: Soft abdomen with uterus appropriate size for dates
Eyes: Normal acuity and visual fields bilaterally
                   Pupils equal and reactive to light
                   Normal eye movements
                   Right eye: normal
                   Left eye: diffuse erythema of sclera; no discharge

Questions

1. What is the differential diagnosis for this woman's red eye?
2. What symptoms should prompt ophthalmological review?
3. What treatment would be appropriate to use in pregnancy?

Answers

1. What is the differential diagnosis for this woman's red eye?

Episcleritis is the most likely diagnosis in this case. Typical symptoms include redness, irritation, and watering of the eyes. Pain is unusual and vision is unaffected. One or both eyes may be affected, and the redness may affect one area of the eye or be more diffuse. Though most often it is idiopathic, it can be associated with systemic conditions such as inflammatory bowel disease, spondyloarthritidies, and some vasculitidies. It usually resolves spontaneously. If patients are irritated by the episcleritis, topical lubricants are first-line therapy. If this is insufficient, topical NSAIDs and/or topical glucocorticoids can be used. Oral NSAIDs can be used prior to 28 weeks of gestation in women with severe or recurrent episcleritis, and oral glucocorticoids may be required in a few resistant cases.

Infective conjunctivitis is also a possibility. The conjunctiva covers the anterior part of the eye and inner surface of the eye lids and conjunctivitis is therefore associated with diffuse erythema of the eye. It can be infective (bacterial or viral) or non-infectious in origin (including allergic or toxic). In addition to redness, there is a crusty discharge which often results in 'sticky' eyes (i.e. difficulty opening the eye lids in the morning). During the day, the discharge is usually clear and stringy in viral and allergic conjunctivitis, and thick and purulent in bacterial conjunctivitis. Infective conjunctivitis is highly contagious, and often the second eye is affected 1–2 days after the first. Bacterial conjunctivitis is often spread from and between children. Viral conjunctivitis usually resolves spontaneously in a few days. Bacterial conjunctivitis can be treated with topical antibiotics.

Anterior uveitis (also known as iritis) is another cause, and redness is usually of the limbus (the junction of the cornea and sclera). It is typically associated with pain and a constricted pupil. There can be some alteration in vision. Women with possible anterior uveitis need urgent ophthalmological review; the diagnosis is confirmed by the presence of leucocytes in the anterior chamber which are visible with a slit-lamp. Topical glucocorticoids are the first-line treatment and dilating drops such as cyclopentolate can relieve the pain.

Bacterial keratitis is a condition from which contact lens wearers are at particular risk. In addition to diffuse erythema, patients complain of a foreign body sensation in the eye, photophobia, and trouble keeping the eye open. There is usually a corneal opacity that can be seen with a pen light, and purulent discharge, which can be mistaken for simple bacterial conjunctivitis. Women at risk of keratitis should have urgent review by an ophthalmologist. Treatment is with topical antibiotics.

2. What symptoms should prompt urgent ophthalmological review?

Most common causes of an acute red eye are either self-limiting (episcleritis, viral conjunctivitis) or can be treated with simple topical antibiotics (bacterial conjunctivitis). However. there are symptoms that should prompt urgent ophthalmological review as they can suggest a potentially sight-threatening condition. These include reduced visual acuity, photophobia, a severe foreign body sensation, particularly one that prevents the person from opening their eye, corneal opacity, severe headache, fixed pupil, or ciliary flush (redness predominantly where the sclera meets the cornea).

3. What treatment would be appropriate to use in pregnancy?

Studies of pregnancies exposed to chloramphenicol showed no increased risk of fetal anomalies. Though data are lacking, the amount of systemic absorption from eye drops is likely to be small, therefore drugs which are known to be safe when used orally are likely to be safe when used as eye drops (e.g. glucocorticoid eye drops). For other medications, the benefits and risks must be considered. Eye drops used for dilatation (tropicamide, phenylephrine, and cyclopentolate) appear safe in pregnancy, though phenylephrine is generally avoided due to potential vasoconstrictive effects. Lidocaine, used as a topical anaesthetic, also appears to be safe.

Further reading

1. Use of eye drops in pregnancy: a monograph. UK Teratology Information Service summary. August 2021. <https://www.medicinesinpregnancy.org/bumps/monographs/USE-OF-EYE-DROPS-IN-PREGNANCY/>

Case 22

A 37-year-old woman attended the Maternity Assessment Unit at 26 weeks of gestation, reporting a 4-day history of itchy feet and arms which was so severe that she could not sleep. There was no associated rash. She initially thought she had been bitten by an insect but there was no evidence of any bites. She reported dark urine but was uncertain about whether her stool was paler in colour than normal. She was in her first pregnancy, and at booking her BP, BMI, and routine bloods were normal. She had no significant past medical history. She was taking vitamin D supplements and had not taken any new medications or supplements in the weeks preceding this presentation. She described allergies to penicillin and peanuts. She did try some chlorphenamine which helped her sleep but did not improve the itch. She worked as a teacher and had never smoked.

Initial assessment

General inspection:	Well
Heart rate:	80 bpm
Blood pressure:	119/67 mmHg
Respiratory rate:	14 breaths/minute
Temperature:	36.6 °C
Oxygen saturations:	99% on room air
Urinalysis:	No protein

Examination

Cardiovascular:	Normal heart sounds, no murmurs
Respiratory:	Normal breath sounds
Abdomen:	Soft and non-tender; no organomegaly; gravid uterus appropriate size for dates.
Skin:	Excoriation on feet, ankles, and arms

Bloods

See Table 22.1.

Table 22.1 Bloods

Haemoglobin	112 g/L
WCC	4.3 × 10⁹/L
Platelets	175 × 10⁹/L
Sodium	137 mmol/L
Potassium	3.7 mmol/L
Urea	2.3 mmol/L
Creatinine	50 μmol/L
Bilirubin	3 μmol/L
ALT	190 iU/L
ALP	162 iU/L
Albumin	29 g/L
Bile acids	134 μmol/L
TSH	2.4 mIU/L
fT4	12.3 pmol/L
Prothrombin time	10.3 secs
APTT	29 s

Questions

1. What are the potential causes of her symptoms?
2. What investigations should be performed in a woman with pruritus in pregnancy?
3. How would you manage this woman's symptoms?

Answers

1. What are the potential causes of her symptoms?

Intrahepatic cholestasis of pregnancy (ICP, commonly known as obstetric cholestasis) is a liver disorder of pregnancy, characterized by pruritus with increased maternal serum bile acids, in the absence of another cause. It affects 0.7% of pregnancies, but higher rates of 1.2–1.5% are found in women from Indian-Asian or Pakistani-Asian origin. Women who have ICP in one pregnancy tend to have recurrence in subsequent pregnancies. The pathophysiology is not understood completely, but there is a genetic component and genes associated with ICP include *ABCB4, BDR3, ATP8B1, ABCB11, ABCC2*, and *Hr1H4*. There is also a hormonal aspect, with the higher levels of oestrogen and progesterone in the second half of pregnancy contributing to cholestasis. Susceptible women may report similar cholestasis when taking the oestrogen-containing oral contraceptive pill.

Itching affecting palms and soles of the feet is characteristic of ICP, but it can occur on any part of the body. In addition to itch, other cholestatic symptoms can occur, including dark urine and pale stool. Jaundice is uncommon. There is no rash in ICP, though there may be associated marks from excoriation.

Pruritus gravidarum is itching without a rash which typically occurs in the third trimester. It can present in a similar way to intrahepatic cholestasis of pregnancy, but liver function tests and bile acids are normal.

Dermatoses of pregnancy can cause diagnostic difficulty in women presenting like this, as there are number of pregnancy-specific rashes which often present with itch. These include atopic eruption of pregnancy, polymorphic eruption of pregnancy, and pemphigoid gestationis (see Case 4).

Atopic dermatitis may flare in pregnancy due to hormonal changes, or due to women stopping their regular emollients/treatment while pregnant.

Allergic or drug reactions can occur at any gestation, presenting with similar symptoms to those in non-pregnant individuals, including a maculopapular rash, and there is likely to be a history of exposure to the offending antigen.

Systemic disease including iron deficiency anaemia, liver, renal, and thyroid disease can all cause pruritus. These may have been diagnosed prior to pregnancy, or other signs/symptoms may be seen in pregnancy.

4. What investigations should be performed in a woman with pruritus in pregnancy?

Routine blood tests
FBC, renal and thyroid function are advised.

Liver function tests
Serum ALT and AST may be significantly raised in ICP but may also reflect other cholestatic liver disorders that can cause pruritus, such as viral hepatitis. There may be a rise in bilirubin but this is uncommon. An increased ALP is common in pregnancy as production of the placental isoenzyme means this is elevated above the

normal non-pregnant reference range in many healthy pregnancies and therefore is often not diagnostically useful.

Bile acids
An increase in serum bile acids may be the only abnormal blood test result, but this can lag behind the development of symptoms.

Markers of liver synthetic function
These include albumin, coagulation parameters, lactate, and glucose. If abnormalities in a number of these are present, it is likely to be that another diagnosis is present rather than ICP. ICP can, however, in a small number of women, cause vitamin K deficiency and coagulation abnormalities which can affect mother and baby.

Other causes of liver dysfunction
To make a diagnosis of ICP, tests should be performed to look for other causes of the abnormalities. These include:

- Viral hepatitis screen (hepatitis A, B, and C, CMV, EBV)
- Autoimmune hepatitis screen (ANA, SMA, anti-LKM-1)
- Abdominal ultrasound to ensure there is no structural abnormality of liver or gallbladder, or gallstones

5. How would you manage this woman's symptoms?

Symptom relief can be offered even during the diagnostic work up to confirm ICP. This includes:

Conservative management
All women should be advised that keeping cool can relieve the itch. This includes environmental changes (loose, cool clothing, sitting by a fan, cool baths, ice packs), and the use of naturally cooling topical treatments, such as aqueous cream with 1–2% menthol, calamine, or aloe vera.

Medications
Antihistamines are safe in pregnancy and can help with itch; mildly sedating antihistamines at night are particularly useful when sleep is affected by the itching.

Ursodeoxycholic acid (UDCA) is a secondary bile acid and has long been used in the treatment of ICP. In some, but not all, women it improves itching symptoms (although this benefit is not statistically significant in randomized controlled trials). A recent meta-analysis suggests that UDCA reduces preterm birth but was underpowered to demonstrate improvement in stillbirth.

Vitamin K is recommended to all women with coagulation parameters consistent with vitamin K deficiency and is often advocated for women with signs of malabsorption given the risk of developing vitamin K deficiency.

This patient goes on to have investigations and no other infective, autoimmune, or structural cause for her symptoms was identified. A diagnosis of ICP was made and she was started on ursodeoxycholic acid. Her itching, ALT, and bile acids improve, but six weeks later (at 32 weeks of gestation) her symptoms have gradually worsened again, and she was on the maximum dose of ursodeoxycholic acid without much symptomatic relief. Her ALT was 180 iu/L and bile acids were 124 μmol/l.

Questions

6. Are there any further treatment options available to her?
7. What complications does ICP cause, and what implication does this have for delivery?

Answers

6. Are there any further treatment options available to her?

Rifampicin is used in treatment of cholestatic conditions outside of pregnancy and has been used in ICP in women with severe disease where the maximum dose of ursodeoxycholic acid is not sufficient, and it is too early in pregnancy to plan an elective birth. It can be beneficial both for maternal symptoms and biochemistry. Women should be warned that bodily secretions such as urine will turn orange in colour, and if they wear contact lenses these may discolour.

7. What complications does ICP cause, and what implication does this have for delivery?

ICP is associated with several adverse fetal outcomes. These include stillbirth, pre-term labour, fetal hypoxia, and meconium-stained amniotic fluid.

The overall stillbirth risk in ICP is 1.5 times that of the population background risk. However, the greatest risk is in those women where the peak total bile acid level is 100 µmol/l or over. In these women, the stillbirth rate increases significantly from 35 weeks of gestation.

Timing of birth will depend on local guidelines, but in those women with bile acids over 100 µmol/l, delivery after the 35th week of pregnancy should be considered. For those with milder ICP, delivery around the 39th week of pregnancy should be considered.

Further reading

1. RCOG: Obstetric cholestasis (Green top guideline No 43, August 2022). <https://www.rcog.org.uk/en/guidelines-research-services/guidelines/gtg43/>
2. C. Ovadia *et al.* Association of adverse perinatal outcomes of intrahepatic cholestasis of pregnancy with biochemical markers: Results of aggregate and individual patient data meta-analyses. The Lancet. 2019; **393**(10174): 899–909.
3. C. Ovadia *et al.* Ursodeoxycholic acid in intrahepatic cholestasis of pregnancy: A systematic review and individual participant data meta-analysis. The Lancet. Gastroenterology & Hepatology. 2021; **6**(7): 547–88.

Case 23

A 45-year-old woman in her second pregnancy presented to the maternity assessment unit at 35 weeks of gestation. She reported flashing lights in her eyes as well as a dark spot in the periphery of her vision. The symptoms started when she woke in the morning and had progressed so that the vision in her left eye was very blurred. She also had a dull frontal headache and a swollen face and ankles. Her first pregnancy 5 years previously was uncomplicated. Her past medical history included type 2 diabetes mellitus and she was taking metformin and insulin in pregnancy as well as aspirin. Her blood pressure at booking had been normal (118/70 mmHg). Home blood pressure monitoring during this pregnancy had not identified any high readings. Her sister had suffered with hypertension in pregnancy, but there was no other family history of note. She was a non-smoker.

Initial assessment

General inspection:	Well in herself, peripheral oedema of legs to mid-calf
Heart rate:	89 bpm
Blood pressure:	190/112 mmHg
Respiratory rate:	15 breaths/min
Temperature:	36.9 °C
Oxygen saturations:	99% on room air
Urinalysis:	3+ protein

Examination

Cardiovascular:	Normal heart sounds, no murmurs
Respiratory:	Normal breath sounds
Abdomen:	Mild epigastric tenderness, non-tender gravid uterus
Cranial nerves:	Visual acuity: right—20/20, left—hand-waving only
	Full range of eye movements, all other cranial nerves normal
Upper limbs:	Normal tone, power, coordination, reflexes, and sensation
Lower limbs:	Normal tone and power, symmetrical knee jerks and downgoing plantars; brisk ankle reflexes and 4 beats of clonus bilaterally; normal coordination and sensation

Bloods

See Table 23.1.

Table 23.1 Bloods

Haemoglobin	109 g/L
WCC	12.0×10^9/L
Platelets	120×10^9/L
Sodium	137 mmol/L
Potassium	3.8 mmol/L
Urea	4 mmol/L
Creatinine	79 µmol/L
Bilirubin	4 µmol/L
ALT	160 iU/L
ALP	110 iU/L
Albumin	35 g/L
CRP	7 mg/L

Questions

1. What are the potential causes of her symptoms?
2. What investigations would you perform?
3. What are the treatment priorities?

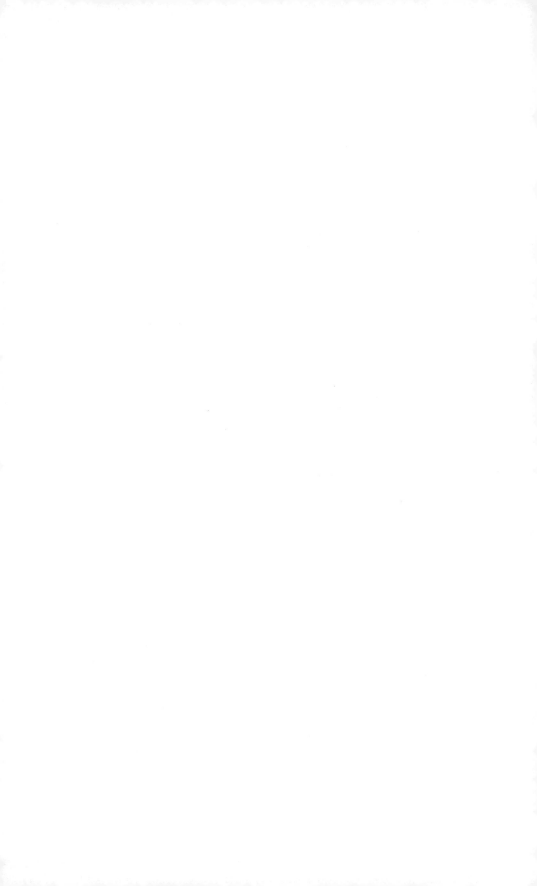

Answers

1. What are the potential causes of her symptoms?

Pre-eclampsia is likely given the new-onset severe hypertension and proteinuria, as well as typical clinical and laboratory features. Pre-eclampsia causes visual disturbance in up to 25% of cases, but this is usually transient and related to hypertension. Visual loss is seen in relatively few cases, so it is important to be vigilant about causes both related to pre-eclampsia and coincident to it.

Retinal detachment occurs when the neurosensory layer of the retina separates from the retinal pigment epithelium and choroid. Serous retinal detachment is rare in pregnancy, affecting 1% of those with severe pre-eclampsia. It is often bilateral.

Cortical blindness is defined as blindness occurring with normal fundoscopy and pupillary function. It is typically a manifestation of PRES and appears to be due to disordered cerebral autoregulation and endothelial dysfunction. In addition to cortical blindness, PRES can cause visual disturbances including visual field defects, headaches, seizures, and altered conscious levels.

Vitreous haemorrhage can occur in the setting of diabetic retinopathy, which can worsen in pregnancy especially in combination with rapid worsening or improvement in glycaemic control. With advanced diabetic retinopathy, new, fragile blood vessels form. These can then rupture, leaking blood as a vitreous haemorrhage. This presents as painless floaters and flashing lights, with the degree of visual loss being proportional to the degree of bleeding. Women with pre-existing diabetes should undergo regular retinal screening to ensure early intervention if any retinal changes are identified.

Central retinal vein or artery occlusion are caused by thrombi in the central retinal vein or artery respectively. Visual field defects vary from scotoma to complete blindness, often with blurred or greyed vision. These develop over hours to weeks and is painless. There may be proceeding scintillations (flashing or flickering). Venous thromboses are more commonly seen particularly in late pregnancy and the postpartum period, related to hypercoagulability. Women with cardiovascular risk factors, such as hypertension and diabetes, are more at risk of arterial thrombi.

Migraine is very common in pregnancy and can occur in women with no history of migraine pre-pregnancy. In women who have previously experienced migraine, the frequency may worsen in pregnancy, but it is also possible for migraine to change in nature. Migraines can be associated with visual disturbance, particularly scintillating scotoma which can give flashing lights and visual obscurations (transient loss of vision). Migrainous aura without headache can also occur.

Central serous chorioretinopathy is a rare condition but occurs a little more commonly in pregnancy. The retina becomes detached due to fluid leak from capillaries within the choroid. The underlying pathophysiology is unknown but is likely to be due to changes in vascular permeability, change in osmotic pressures, and changes in prostaglandin levels. It can present as blurred vision, micropsia (images appear smaller), or metamorphosia (images are distorted).

Acute angle-closure glaucoma can manifest as blurred vision and visual loss, however, the other symptoms such as headaches, severe eye pain, eye redness, and seeing haloes around lights are absent in this case which makes the diagnosis less likely.

2. What investigations would you perform?

This woman is acutely unwell, and the priority should be to stabilize her and manage her pre-eclampsia both medically and plan birth. Once she is stabilized, she should undergo:

Fundoscopy at the bedside as this will allow gross retinal detachment or haemorrhage to be seen.

Formal ophthalmological assessment to assess the pupil and the retina thoroughly using tools such as slit-lamp assessment and optical coherence tomography.

MRI brain should be performed if no pupillary or retinal disease is found. Pathology such as PRES may be identified this way.

3. What are the treatment priorities?

The priority is to stabilize her and optimize treatment of pre-eclampsia. This will involve medications to treat her blood pressure such as oral labetalol or modified release nifedipine, or intravenous labetalol or hydralazine. Intravenous magnesium sulphate is indicated to reduce the occurrence of eclamptic seizures. Once stabilized, a delivery plan can be made.

Fetal assessment with CTG is important as urgent birth would only be required if there was evidence of acute fetal compromise, otherwise the antihypertensive treatment would be optimized as an inpatient, and delivery undertaken when indicated by the maternal or fetal condition.

Vaginal delivery in pre-eclampsia can be considered if her clinical condition is stabilized and there are no other obstetric factors.

Ocular conditions such as myopia, retinal detachment, and vitreous haemorrhage are not contra-indications to vaginal birth as there is no evidence that labour and the Valsalva manoeuvre alter vitreous pressure.

Cortical blindness and retinal detachment due to pre-eclampsia should be managed conservatively as these are likely to resolve as the pre-eclampsia resolves.

Vitreous haemorrhage, retinal detachment, and retinal vein or artery occlusions need to be treated within specialist ophthalmic services. Retinal photocoagulation and intra-ophthalmic injections of steroids or anti-VEGF may all be used in pregnancy.

Further reading

1. H. Chiu *et al.* Delivery recommendations for pregnant females with risk factors for rhegmatogenous retinal detachment. Canadian Journal of Ophthalmology. 2015; **50**(1): 11–18.
2. A. Patil *et al.* Ocular manifestations of pregnancy and labour: From the innocuous to the sight threatening. The Obstetrician and Gynaecologist. 2020; **22**(3): 217–26.

Case 24

A 32-year-old woman called the maternity advice line when she was 26 weeks pregnant. She was concerned as she worked as a primary school teacher and one of the children in her class had developed a rash which looked like chickenpox. The patient had not had chickenpox as a child and had not been vaccinated. She had been feeling well throughout pregnancy and had no similar symptoms.

This was her second pregnancy; her first pregnancy had been uncomplicated, and she had delivered vaginally at term. She was taking pregnancy multivitamins but no regular medication. She was a non-smoker and did not drink alcohol.

Questions

1. What are the possible consequences of varicella-zoster exposure in pregnancy?
2. What treatment would you offer at this stage in pregnancy?
3. What treatment would you offer her if she develops a chickenpox rash?

Answers

1. What are the possible consequences of varicella-zoster exposure in pregnancy?

Primary infection with varicella-zoster virus (VZV) in pregnancy can affect both mother and fetus. It is spread by direct contact with vesicles, saliva, or the mucus of an infected person, as well as through aerosol droplets from coughing and sneezing.

Uncomplicated varicella infection is characterized by a vesicular rash, which appears in clusters over the face, trunk, and limbs over a number of days. There may be a prodrome of myalgia, fever, and malaise 1–4 days prior to the rash. The rash appears as macules, then papules, and then vesicles, which then become pustular and then crust over. Most people have crops of lesions at different stages for a few days, though usually by day 6, all lesions have crusted over. The crusts tend to resolve within 1–2 weeks and may leave a hypopigmented area.

Pregnant women are at risk of more severe VZV infection. This can include pneumonia most commonly, but also neurological infection (meningitis, encephalitis, and cerebellar ataxia), hepatitis, glomerulonephritis, myocarditis, ocular disease, adrenal insufficiency, and death. There may also be secondary bacterial infection of the skin lesions.

Varicella pneumonia presents with cough, dyspnoea, rash, and tachypnoea, usually within 1 week of the rash. There may be a diffuse miliary infiltrate on the chest radiography, which is usually bilateral. The clinical course is variable, but significant hypoxia and respiratory failure can occur.

Depending on the gestation, primary infection of the mother can cause fetal varicella syndrome (FVS, also known as congenital varicella syndrome). Infection in the second trimester carries the greatest risk, particularly between 13 and 20 weeks of gestation. FVS is characterized by intrauterine growth restriction, cutaneous scars in a dermatomal pattern, neurological defects including intellectual disability, hydrocephaly, microcephaly, cortical atrophy, or ventriculomegaly, seizures and Horner's syndrome, ocular problems such as optic nerve atrophy, cataracts, and chorioretinitis, limb abnormalities such as hypoplasia, atrophy and paresis, and gastrointestinal problems including reflux, and atretic or stenotic bowel. FVS is associated with 30% mortality in the first 3 months of life and a 15% risk of shingles in the first 4 years of life. Transmission rates are fortunately low; whilst viral DNA is detected in the amniotic fluid of 8% of women with infection during pregnancy, the incidence of FVS is 0.91%.

If the woman is infected in the 4 weeks prior to delivery, there is a 1 in 4 risk of infection in the neonate. The highest risk is if infection is within 2–5 days of childbirth as maternal IgG has not developed and passed to the infant. Varicella of the neonate can range from a mild illness with a rash and fever to a disseminated infection like that seen in immunocompromised individuals, with pneumonia, meningoencephalitis, and hepatitis.

Unlike primary VZV infection, reactivation of latent VZV (herpes zoster or 'shingles') is not associated with significant FVS.

2. What treatment would you offer at this stage in pregnancy?

The initial step is establishing the degree of exposure to the virus. If the contact with an infected individual is not face to face, and is for less than 15 minutes, it is not considered significant. If a woman has a clear history of previous varicella infection, she can also be reassured. This woman had a significant exposure and no history of infection, so varicella antibodies should be checked urgently. This can be done either by using the serum sample, which was saved when booking bloods were taken, or a sample taken at the time of presentation. Many people without prior history are found to have antibodies. Varicella zoster immunoglobulin (VZIG) can be given to all non-immune and non-vaccinated pregnant women exposed to VZV. It should be given as soon as possible after VZV exposure but is efficacious up to 10 days after contact with the infected person. If there is further exposure to varicella, a second dose of VZIG can be given 3 weeks after the first dose.

Women who receive VZIG should be treated as potentially infectious from 8–28 days after exposure, which includes avoiding contact with other potentially non-immune pregnant women during that time.

All pregnant women should inform the healthcare professionals managing their pregnancy so that appropriate action can be taken if the woman becomes un-well, and so that appropriate isolation procedures can be put in place if she needs assistance.

3. What treatment would you offer her if she develops a chickenpox rash?

Oral aciclovir is suggested for pregnant women with uncomplicated varicella over 20 weeks of gestation and can be considered prior to 20 weeks of gestation. Women should be informed that aciclovir is not licensed in pregnancy, but there is no evidence of an increased rate of congenital anomalies. Oral aciclovir is most efficacious if started within 24 hours of symptoms.

All pregnant women with severe infection, including varicella pneumonia or central nervous system infection, should be treated with intravenous aciclovir, with antibiotics if there is concern about a superadded bacterial infection.

All women with a varicella rash should stay away from other vulnerable people (including other pregnant women) until the rash has completely crusted over.

Women who develop varicella infection in pregnancy should be seen by a fetal medicine specialist to discuss the risks of fetal varicella infection and arrange additional ultrasound examinations if appropriate. Amniocentesis can be performed to look for varicella DNA in the amniotic fluid. This invasive sampling carries a 1% risk of miscarriage. Ultrasound and amniocentesis have a good negative predictive value for excluding FVS but have poor positive predictive value. The neonatal team should be informed of any woman who develops varicella during pregnancy so they can arrange appropriate review and testing of the baby.

If possible, planned birth should be delayed until at least 7 days after the start of the infection to allow passive transfer of maternal antibodies and reduce the risk of varicella infection of the neonate. In addition, birth during active infection be associated with coagulopathy and/or haemorrhage due to hepatitis or thrombo- cytopenia. The method of birth should be determined on a case-by-case basis. If neuraxial anaesthesia is used, there is a risk of transmission of virus from the skin to the central nervous system. Epidural anaesthesia may be safer than spinal an- aesthesia as it avoids dural puncture. Postpartum, women with varicella can be reassured that it is safe for them to breastfeed.

Further reading

1. RCOG: Chickenpox in Pregnancy (Green top Guideline No 13, 2015). <https://www.rcog.org. uk/globalassets/documents/guidelines/gtg13.pdf>

Case 25

A 21-year-old woman with type 1 diabetes mellitus attended the obstetric diabetes clinic at 35 weeks of gestation. She reported that she had been woken by the alarm on her continuous glucose monitor on four occasions over the last week due to early morning hypoglycaemia. She had also had two hypoglycaemic episodes during the day over the last 2 days, despite a reduction in basal insulin rate on her pump over the last week.

She had had some hypoglycaemic episodes in the first trimester, but her glucose control had stabilized in the second trimester. She had gradually increased her total daily insulin dosage as pregnancy progressed. Her last growth scan at 32 weeks of gestation had shown a fetus with an estimated fetal weight over the 50th centile with normal liquor and normal umbilical artery Dopplers.

Her insulin was delivered by an insulin pump (containing insulin aspart), and she was taking regular aspirin and vitamin D. Her HbA1c at the start of pregnancy was 53 mmol/mol and was 49 mmol/mol at 28 weeks of gestation. She had no other medical conditions.

Initial assessment

General inspection:	Well
Heart rate:	96 bpm
Blood pressure:	142/89 mmHg
Respiratory rate:	14 breaths/minute
Temperature:	36.8 °C
Oxygen saturations:	99% on room air
Urinalysis:	No protein, glucose, or ketones

Examination

Cardiovascular:	Normal heart sounds
Respiratory:	Normal breath sounds throughout
Abdomen:	Soft and non-tender

Bloods

See Table 25.1.

Table 25.1 Bloods

Haemoglobin	121 g/L
WCC	7.32 × 10⁹/L
Platelets	273 × 10⁹/L
Sodium	138 mmol/L
Potassium	4.2 mmol/L
Urea	2.5 mmol/L
Creatinine	55 μmol/L
Bilirubin	9 μmol/L
ALT	11 iU/L
ALP	68 iU/L
Albumin	34 g/L
CRP	6 mg/L

A repeat fetal growth scan showed a reduction in growth velocity, with the estimated fetal weight under the 20th centile. The decision was made to induce labour.

Questions

1. What is the role of continuous glucose monitoring in pregnancy?
2. What is the role of an insulin pump in pregnancy?
3. What are the causes of hypoglycaemia in pregnancy?
4. How should this woman's blood glucose be controlled during her induction and labour?
5. What changes should be made to her insulin dose after delivery?

Answers

1. When should continuous glucose monitoring be used in pregnancy?

The National Institute for Health and Clinical Excellence recommends that continuous glucose monitoring (CGM) is offered to all women with type 1 diabetes during pregnancy. Flash glucose monitoring can also be offered to women with type 1 diabetes who cannot use CGM or prefer flash monitoring.

Continuous and flash glucose monitors are both devices worn on the skin and measure interstitial fluid glucose levels. This means they can produce slightly different results compared to capillary blood glucose levels, but work without the need for finger pricking. CGM continuously transmits data about interstitial glucose levels to a receiver device which can be read by the user at any point, whereas flash monitoring only gives a reading when the device on the skin is scanned. Both devices give predictions about whether blood glucose is going up or down, provide information about blood glucose patterns, and have alarms that warn about both high and low blood glucose levels. Historically CGM has been more accurate at low blood glucose levels so is preferred in patients with a history of severe hypoglycaemic episodes, but the technology is continually improving and rapidly developing.

CGM can also be considered in women on insulin therapy with type 2 diabetes or gestational diabetes if they have problematic, severe hypoglycaemia, or unstable blood glucose levels that are causing concern despite efforts to optimize glycaemic control.

In pregnant women with type 1 diabetes CGM has been shown to increase the time spent in the target blood sugar range, reduce the risk of large-for-gestational age babies, reduce neonatal hypoglycaemia and neonatal intensive care admissions, and reduce the length of hospital stay.

2. Who should use a continuous subcutaneous insulin infusion (CSII or insulin pump) in pregnancy?

Increasing numbers of women with type 1 diabetes use a continuous subcutaneous insulin infusion (CSII) outside pregnancy, either to improve glycaemic control or because of disabling hypoglycaemia. There is no evidence that CSII improves pregnancy outcomes, and there are some study data suggesting the use of CSII is associated with an increased risk of gestational hypertension, neonatal hypoglycaemia, and neonatal intensive care admission. CSII therapy should therefore be continued on women already established on it prior to pregnancy but it should only be started in pregnancy in exceptional circumstances.

Placental hormones and cytokines cause insulin resistance, so insulin doses in type 1 diabetes increase gradually throughout pregnancy and the pump settings will require regular review and adjustment.

3. What are the possible causes of hypoglycaemia in this woman?

A physiological fall in insulin resistance can occur in some women, without associated adverse outcomes.

Placental insufficiency may cause a drop in insulin resistance and therefore in the insulin doses required to maintain good glycaemic control. Other indicators of placental insufficiency such as reduced growth velocity or markers of pre-eclampsia may also occur. This can be hard to distinguish from a physiological fall in insulin resistance, but pre-eclampsia is more common in women with a fall in daily insulin requirements of 15% or more. In this case, the fall in growth velocity and borderline elevated systolic blood pressure suggest there is placental insufficiency, which may be the cause of hypoglycaemia.

Placental insufficiency may also contribute to the increased risk of stillbirth in women with pre-existing diabetes. However, placental insufficiency secondary to diabetes may be difficult to diagnose. Women with a significant fall in daily insulin requirements and/or unexplained hypoglycaemia in late pregnancy must therefore be assessed by experienced clinicians, and delivery expedited if there is a concern about placental failure.

Acute fatty liver of pregnancy can present with hypoglycaemia whether or not the woman has diabetes, but it would be unusual for this to be the only abnormality at presentation.

Other systemic conditions such as cortisol deficiency, liver failure, malaria, or severe sepsis can result in hypoglycaemia. No other markers of these conditions were seen in this woman.

Hypoglycaemia is common in early pregnancy in women with diabetes, with more than 45% of women experiencing severe hypoglycaemia (defined as hypoglycaemia that requires third-party assistance to treat). Previous severe hypoglycaemic episodes and hypoglycaemic unawareness are risk factors for this. Nausea and vomiting in pregnancy are not risk factors for hypoglycaemia. Hypoglycaemia can cause significant maternal morbidity and mortality; however the fetal effects of hypoglycaemia are unknown.

4. How should this woman's blood glucose be controlled during her induction and labour?

Variable rate intravenous insulin infusions (VRIII) are used in many women with type 1 diabetes during labour to maintain good glycaemic control. Women who use CSII, however, and who feel confident in managing their pump during labour and birth, can continue to use their pump if they wish. Insulin requirements drop rapidly during labour, therefore prior to labour a temporary basal rate should be programmed into the CSII (e.g. 50% of the basal rate), with correction doses administered to treat hyperglycaemia. If there are difficulties in managing the CSII at any time, a VRIII should be started.

Good glycaemic control in labour can reduce the risk of diabetic ketoacidosis or unexpected hypoglycaemia, however it does not reduce rates of neonatal hypoglycaemia or reduce neonatal intensive care unit admissions.

Administration of steroids for fetal lung maturation often causes hyperglycaemia, even in women without diabetes. In women with diabetes, this hyperglycaemia may require additional treatment such as a VRIII, or adjustments to their CSII settings, for 24–48 hours.

5. What changes should be made to her insulin dose after delivery?

Women with diabetes are at high risk of hypoglycaemia in the postpartum period, especially for the 24–48 hours after birth. This occurs as insulin resistance drops after delivery of the placenta, and metabolic demands change, particularly with breastfeeding. Once eating and drinking, women should restart their normal insulin (either multiple daily injections or CSII), but at approximately 60–75% of the pre-pregnancy dose. Capillary blood glucose levels should be checked regularly, and hypoglycaemia treated appropriately with oral or intravenous glucose alongside long-acting carbohydrate.

Further reading

1. Diabetes in pregnancy: Management from preconception to the postnatal period. (NICE guideline No 3, last updated 16 December 2020). <https://www.nice.org.uk/guidance/ng3>
2. **D. Feig** *et al.* Continuous glucose monitoring in pregnant women with type 1 diabetes (CONCEPTT): A multicentre international randomised controlled trial. The Lancet. 2017; **390**(10110): 2347–59.

Case 26

A 36-year-old woman in her second pregnancy presented at 25 weeks of gestation with shortness of breath and lethargy. She also reported headache, visual disturbances, and feeling dizzy. Her pregnancy had been complicated by protracted nausea and vomiting beyond the first trimester, severely limiting her oral intake. Anaemia had been identified on her booking bloods and she had been treated with oral iron. Her first pregnancy had also been complicated by nausea and vomiting throughout pregnancy, and she had an uncomplicated vaginal birth at term.

Initial assessment

General inspection: Well in herself, pale
Heart rate: 98 bpm
Blood pressure: 115/76 mmHg
Temperature: 36.1 °C
Oxygen saturations: 98%
Urinalysis: 3+ protein

Examination

Cardiovascular: Normal
Respiratory: Normal
Abdomen: Soft, non-tender gravid uterus
Neurological: Normal examination

Bloods

See Table 26.1.

Table 26.1 Bloods

Haemoglobin	58 g/L
MCV	106 fL
WCC	2.6 × 10⁹/L
Platelets	110 × 10⁹/L
Sodium	136 mmol/L
Potassium	2.7 mmol/L
Urea	2.2 mmol/L
Creatinine	50 μmol/L
Bilirubin	5 μmol/L
ALT	10 iU/L
ALP	100 iU/L
Albumin	28 g/L
CRP	5 mg/L
LDH	4532 IU/L
Ferritin	35 mcg/L
B12	120 ng/L
Folate	< 3 mcg/L

Questions

1. What are the possible causes for this presentation?
2. What are the causes for macrocytosis in pregnancy?
3. What management would you recommend for the most likely diagnosis?
4. What are the risks to mother and baby?

Answers

1. What are the possible causes for this presentation?

She has pancytopenia, with macrocytic red cells and a very elevated LDH, suggestive of haemolysis. She also has new proteinuria.

Folate deficiency is rare outside pregnancy, but common during pregnancy due to increasing folate requirements of up to 800 micrograms per day (attributable to high fetal demand and increased red cell mass) as compared to 50–400 micrograms in non-pregnant women. Risk factors for folate deficiency include poor dietary intake and malabsorption syndromes such as coeliac disease and Crohn's disease. It is important to have a low threshold for asking about dietary intake and assessing risk factors for folate deficiency. Transient proteinuria in the setting of severe folate deficiency has been observed, but the mechanism is unclear.

B12 deficiency takes longer to develop, and so is much less likely to present *de novo* in pregnancy. B12 stores take longer to deplete compared to folate, and the normal range in pregnancy is lower than the normal reference range used in non-pregnant adults. This may mean there is clinical uncertainty about whether a low B12 result represents true B12 deficiency. However, deficiency of B12 and folate may coexist and contribute to the megaloblastic anaemia. There is a risk that folate replacement alone can precipitate subacute combined degeneration of the cord if B12 deficiency is present and untreated, so it is appropriate to replace B12 alongside folate in women who develop complications of haematinic deficiency. Tests including methylmalonic acid (MMA) and homocysteine can be helpful if there is clinical suspicion of B12 deficiency but the levels of B12 are not diagnostic (MMA and homocysteine increase in B12 deficiency, homocysteine alone increases in folate deficiency).

Haemolysis, elevated liver enzymes and low platelets (HELLP) is suggested by the possible haemolysis and low platelets, but her liver function tests are normal. She has new proteinuria which is also suggestive of a hypertensive disorder of pregnancy but is normotensive on presentation. Hypertension and/or proteinuria may be absent in HELLP, so HELLP is still possible in this case.

Thrombotic thrombocytopenic purpura must be considered whenever there is a suggestion of a microangiopathic haemolytic anaemia and low platelets. Rapid diagnosis and institution of treatment such as plasma exchange are crucial in this condition. However, severe folate deficiency can result in fragmentation of red cells, which may confuse the clinical picture when identified on the blood film. In addition, haemolysis itself can lead to folate depletion. This all means that a careful clinical assessment and early use of other tests such as ADAMTS-13 are crucial.

2. What are other possible causes for a macrocytosis in pregnancy?

The causes of a macrocytic anaemia can be divided into megaloblastic (folate and B12 deficiency described above) and non-megaloblastic. Non-megaloblastic causes include hypothyroidism, a high reticulocyte count, alcohol intake, some medications, and myelodysplasia, but can occasionally be seen as a result of pregnancy alone, with no underlying cause identified.

3. What management would you recommend for the most likely diagnosis?

A blood film is a crucial test and may confirm the diagnosis if classic changes of megaloblastic anaemia are seen (macrocytic red cells, although this can be masked if concurrent iron deficiency is also present, hypersegmented neutrophils, reduction in reticulocytes, the presence of Howell–Jolly bodies). Changes of haemolysis may also be present, as discussed above.

Folate replacement is easy to do and has a rapid effect, and despite the severity of the anaemia, she does not necessarily require blood products. High-dose oral folic acid (5 mg up to three times daily) leads to rapid repletion of folate levels and an increase in haemoglobin should be seen within days of initiation.

B12 replacement should be undertaken if there are clinical signs or symptoms of B12 deficiency, or megaloblastic changes on the blood film.

Oral thiamine should be considered if there is concern about the duration of poor oral intake and risk of vitamin deficiency.

Oral iron can be given as her ferritin levels are not high, and it is likely that the demand for iron increases as erythrocytosis increases in response to folate and B12 replacement.

Consideration of the cause is an important part of the management, for example addressing and treating significant nausea and vomiting, as well as looking for evidence of malabsorption for example tissue transglutaminase antibodies for coeliac disease.

A blood film showed changes consistent with folate deficiency (macrocytosis and hypersegmented neutrophils). Treatment including oral folic acid 5 mg three times daily, intramuscular B12, oral ferrous sulphate, and oral thiamine was started. Response to treatment was confirmed by changes on repeated blood films and haemoglobin. She experienced a rapid improvement in her symptoms and her haemoglobin had increased to 115 g/L prior to birth. Her proteinuria also resolved after folate replacement.

Question

4. What are the risks to the baby?

Answer

4. What are the risks to the baby?

Several studies have shown the importance of folic acid supplementation pre-conception to prevent, and reduce the recurrence of, neural tube defects. However, the consequences to the fetus from maternal folate deficiency in later pregnancy are not clear. Older studies report an association with increased risk of perinatal morbidity and mortality including stillbirth and placental abruption though the evidence is weak. In common with other causes of maternal anaemia, more recent studies have also demonstrated increased risk of low birthweight and preterm birth.

Case 27

A 19-year-old woman in her first pregnancy was seen urgently in the antenatal clinic. She was approximately 12 weeks pregnant. Nine months prior to conception she had been diagnosed with moderate pulmonary arterial hypertension after extensive investigation and assessment. She had been started on a calcium channel blocker.

She was able to walk up one flight of stairs without stopping but would be short of breath at the top. She became breathless when walking fast. She was World Health Organization (WHO) functional class II. She did not have any orthopnoea or paroxysmal dyspnoea, and no cough. She reported ankle swelling, particularly at night. She complained of worsening fatigue and dull substernal chest discomfort and occasional light-headedness.

She had no other past medical history. She did not drink alcohol or smoke cigarettes.

Examination

General inspection:	GCS 15/15, no central cyanosis
Heart rate:	102 beats per minute, regular
Blood pressure:	110/60 mmHg
Respiratory rate:	18 breaths/minute
Temperature:	36.9 °C
Oxygen saturations:	93% on room air
Urinalysis:	No protein

Examination

Cardiovascular:	Elevated jugular venous pressure, fourth heart sound, right ventricular heave
Respiratory:	Reduced air entry at both bases
Abdominal:	No organomegaly; uterus appropriate size for gestation

Bloods

See Table 27.1.

Table 27.1 Bloods

Haemoglobin	131 g/L
WCC	6.32 × 10⁹/L
Platelets	273 × 10⁹/L
Sodium	138 mmol/L
Potassium	4.2 mmol/L
Urea	5 mmol/L
Creatinine	55 µmol/L
Bilirubin	7 µmol/L
ALT	12 iU/L
Albumin	30 g/L
CRP	6 mg/L

Questions

1. Why does pulmonary hypertension cause cardiovascular compromise in pregnancy?
2. What complications are associated with pulmonary hypertension in pregnancy?
3. What investigations should she have during pregnancy?
4. What treatment is appropriate in pregnancy?
5. What mode and timing of delivery should be advised?
6. What contraception would you offer this woman at the end of pregnancy?

Answers

1. Why does pulmonary hypertension cause cardiovascular compromise in pregnancy?

In normal pregnancy there is an increase in plasma volume, systemic vasodilation, and a reduction in systemic vascular resistance, which leads to an increase in cardiac output. In women with pulmonary arterial hypertension, however, the pulmonary vasculature is unable to dilate and accommodate the higher pulmonary blood flow, resulting in a rise in pulmonary artery pressure and limitation of cardiac output. The right ventricle dilates and both systolic and diastolic dysfunction may occur. There may also be reduced right coronary perfusion pressure, which can lead to right ventricular ischaemia. Overall this significantly compromises cardiac function.

2. What are the complications associated with pulmonary hypertension in pregnancy?

Risks to the mother

Maternal mortality of up to 33% is reported if pulmonary hypertension is severe, though more typically is reported in the range of 9–25%. As the disease can worsen in pregnancy, there is no level of pulmonary hypertension which is considered safe in pregnancy. Death is usually due to pulmonary hypertension crises, venous thromboembolism, or right heart failure. This is most common in the third trimester or early in the postpartum period. Due to the risk of maternal death, pulmonary artery hypertension is in the modified World Health Organization Class IV for maternal cardiovascular risk, where it is advised that pregnancy and fertility treatment should be avoided.

Heart failure may occur, particularly right-sided heart failure, as right ventricular function is compromised in pregnancy.

Atrial arrhythmias may result from atrial enlargement and can occur at any time. As these are poorly tolerated in pregnancy and can be life-threatening, they should be aggressively managed, ideally with rhythm control.

Thromboembolic disease including paradoxical emboli can occur, so anticoagulation should be reviewed in all women.

Hypoxaemia can worsen and is multifactorial, resulting from left-to-right shunting, reduced cardiac output, and diaphragmatic splinting due to the gravid uterus.

Risks to the fetus

Stillbirth or neonatal death occurs in up to 30% of women with pulmonary arterial hypertension, particularly if maternal hypoxia or reduced maternal cardiac output are present, or preterm birth is necessitated.

Intrauterine growth restriction can occur, due to utero-placental hypoxia and ischaemia due to impaired blood flow. In women with cyanotic heart disease, fetal outcomes are better if oxygen saturations are over 90%; saturations below 85% are associated with an increased risk of growth restriction, intrauterine fetal death, and prematurity.

3. What specific investigations should this woman have during pregnancy?

Specific blood tests include BNP which should be measured at the first visit, and at least monthly, as this may help identify right ventricular failure.

An ECG at the first visit is helpful, as well as whenever symptoms or concerns arise, due to the risks of arrhythmias.

Echocardiography should be performed regularly during pregnancy and used to monitor cardiac function including left ventricular ejection fraction, right ventricular overload, and pulmonary artery pressures.

Fetal ultrasound to assess fetal growth is required to assess for intrauterine growth restriction. A fetal echocardiogram is also recommended at 20–24 weeks of gestation in women with pulmonary hypertension in the setting of congenital heart disease.

4. How should this woman be managed in pregnancy?

Due to the significant risks of pulmonary arterial hypertension in pregnancy, all women must be managed by a multidisciplinary team including experts in both maternal and fetal medicine, pulmonary hypertension, and cardiac/obstetric anaesthetics. Women should be seen regularly in pregnancy, with monthly review in the first and second trimester, increasing to every 1–2 weeks in the third trimester. Women may need to be admitted to hospital for bed rest to avoid cardiovascular compromise.

Women with pulmonary hypertension are discouraged from becoming pregnant due to the maternal and fetal risks. It is therefore appropriate to discuss a termination of pregnancy with all women with pulmonary hypertension. If the woman opts for a termination, this should be performed at a centre that cares for patients with pulmonary hypertension as the procedure itself carries a risk to the mother.

Specific treatment for pulmonary arterial hypertension can be used in pregnancy, including phosphodiesterase inhibitors and prostacyclin agonists. Calcium channel blockers can be used in the subset of women who are truly responsive to vasodilators. Endothelin receptor antagonists and guanylate cyclase stimulators are teratogenic, so are generally advised against in pregnancy, but there may be some cases where the risk of omitting them outweighs the fetal risks and therefore they are continued or commenced in pregnancy.

Anticoagulation should be continued during pregnancy if the woman is on lifelong anticoagulation when not pregnant, and this is usually changed to LMWH. Prophylactic anticoagulation should be considered for women who are not on anticoagulation prior to pregnancy, due to the increased risk of venous thromboembolism. However, this should be considered on an individual basis due to the risk of bleeding in some cases, particularly in women with Eisenmenger's syndrome, where there is an increased risk of thrombocytopenia and clotting factor deficiency.

Aspirin should be started from 12 weeks of gestation to reduce the risk of pre-eclampsia.

Iron supplementation to correct iron-deficiency anaemia will also help with hypoxaemia and is likely to have a beneficial effect on pulmonary pressures.

Diuretics should be used if there are signs of heart failure and furosemide is first line.

5. What mode and timing of delivery should be advised?

The mode and timing of birth must be considered on an individual basis. It is often suggested that women should give birth between 34 and 37 weeks of gestation. Pulmonary hypertension is not an absolute contra-indication to vaginal birth. However, during contractions there is a substantial autotransfusion of blood from the uterus into the mother's circulation, and immediately postpartum there is a 60–80% increase in cardiac output due to shifts in blood from the uterus to the maternal circulation, mobilization of extravascular fluid, and the inferior vena cava no longer being compressed by the gravid uterus. The timing of birth also influences the advice about delivery method. A caesarean section does not mitigate all the risks of delivery but may allow these to be managed in an optimally controlled way. Whether a vaginal or caesarean delivery is chosen, an experienced obstetric/cardiac anaesthetist should be present. Neuraxial anaesthesia may be preferred to avoid the cardiovascular stress from the pain of labour, and the cardiovascular changes that occur during general anaesthesia.

The location for postnatal care should also be considered in advance of birth, as these women have a high chance of deterioration in the days after birth and therefore a high dependency unit or intensive care unit is usually appropriate. A negative fluid balance is the aim, with some centres advocating very significant diuresis in the first few days after birth.

6. What contraception would you offer this woman after pregnancy?

Contraception should be discussed with all women with pulmonary arterial hypertension. Long-acting reversible progesterone-only contraceptive methods such as the subdermal implant or depot injection are safe and effective. Hormonal or non-hormonal intrauterine devices are also appropriate and very effective but should be inserted in hospital because of the risk of a vasovagal episode relating to cervical stimulation, which can be poorly tolerated. The combined contraceptive pill should be avoided due the increased risk of thromboembolism. Barrier contraception should not be recommended due to the high failure rate.

Further reading

1. V. **Regitz-Zagrosek** *et al.* 2018 ESC Guidelines for the management of cardiovascular diseases during pregnancy: The Task Force for the Management of Cardiovascular Diseases during Pregnancy of the European Society of Cardiology (ESC) European Heart Journal. 2018; **39**: 3165–241.

2. ESC Guidelines for the management of cardiovascular diseases during pregnancy. European Heart Journal. 2018; https://www.escardio.org/Guidelines/Clinical-Practice-Guidelines/Cardiovascular-Diseases-during-Pregnancy-Management-of

3. **S. Krishnan** *et al*. Pulmonary Hypertension Complicating Pregnancy. Current Pulmonology Reports. 2021; **10**:71–83.

Case 28

A 41-year-old woman was seen in the maternal medicine clinic at 20 weeks of gestation. She was being reviewed regularly due to a background history of Crohn's disease for which she took azathioprine. Ten years prior to pregnancy she had had small bowel obstruction with subsequent laparotomy and ileal resection. Her last flare was 18 months prior, and she had previously had a perianal fistula, but this had healed. At this appointment she described feeling generally unwell, with extreme fatigue, loss of appetite, and had lost 8 kg of weight unintentionally in the preceding few weeks. She described intermittent diarrhoea and constipation, intermittent abdominal pain but no blood or mucus in the stool and no vomiting.

In addition to her regular azathioprine she was also taking omeprazole and vitamin D. She had no other significant medical history. She had never smoked.

Initial assessment

General inspection:	Pale, unwell
Heart rate:	105 bpm
Blood pressure:	110/55 mmHg
Temperature:	37.2 °C
Oxygen saturations:	100% on room air
Urinalysis:	No protein

Examination

Cardiovascular:	Normal heart sounds, no added sounds
Respiratory:	Normal breath sounds
Abdomen:	Diffuse tenderness, worse in the right lower quadrant; normal bowel sounds.
Rectal examination:	No blood or mucus

Bloods

See Table 28.1.

Table 28.1 Bloods

Haemoglobin	108 g/L
WCC	6.32×10^9/L
Platelets	273×10^9/L
Sodium	138 mmol/L
Potassium	4.2 mmol/L
Urea	5 mmol/L
Creatinine	65 µmol/L
Bilirubin	12 µmol/L
ALT	68 iU/L
ALP	110 iU/L
Albumin	24 g/L
CRP	20 mg/L

Questions

1. What are the potential causes for her symptoms?
2. What investigations would you arrange?
3. What treatment would you offer to treat her current symptoms?
4. What treatments can be used to treat inflammatory bowel disease in pregnancy?
5. What are the risks associated with inflammatory bowel disease in pregnancy?
6. What mode of delivery should be recommended for this woman?

Answers

1. What are the potential causes for her symptoms?

A flare of Crohn's disease is the most likely cause of this woman's symptoms given her history. One-third of women with Crohn's disease will have a flare of disease activity in pregnancy or the postpartum period. The symptoms can be non-specific and extraintestinal manifestations such as erythema nodosum, mouth ulcers, or arthritis may occur. The systemic symptoms overlap with some of the normal symptoms of pregnancy. Inflammatory bowel disease is most commonly seen in individuals of reproductive age, so it can present for the first time in pregnancy and should be considered in pregnant women presenting with abdominal symptoms, particularly a change in bowel habit.

Gastrointestinal infection can mimic a flare of Crohn's disease. *Clostridium difficile* infection can cause a pseudomembranous colitis that has similar symptoms and should be considered in women who have had recurrent courses of antibiotics or are otherwise immunocompromised.

Acute appendicitis is diagnosed in approximately 1 in 1000 pregnancies, most commonly in the second trimester. Pregnant women are less likely to present with pain in the classic right iliac fossa location, as the gravid uterus displaces the appendix away from the abdominal wall. Pain may therefore be non-specific, periumbilical, right lower quadrant, right flank, and even right upper quadrant. Systemic symptoms such as nausea, vomiting, heartburn, and malaise can all be mistaken for the typical symptoms of pregnancy.

Malignancy, particularly colorectal cancer, can present in this way. Though colorectal cancer is rare in pregnancy (less than 1 case per 100,000 pregnancies), it is more likely to be diagnosed late and at an advanced stage in pregnancy. It should therefore be considered in any woman presenting with chronic abdominal symptoms and/or unexplained systemic symptoms such as weight loss.

2. What investigations would you arrange?

Blood tests including FBC, renal function, liver function, and CRP are baseline tests in any woman with these symptoms.

Stool samples should be sent for both microbiological assessment and calprotectin. A high level of the latter is a very sensitive marker of bowel inflammation.

Imaging may be required, including abdominal X-ray (rarely indicated in pregnancy, but can be considered if obstruction or inflammation is a concern), ultrasound of small bowel, MRI, or endoscopy.

Oesophageal gastroduodenoscopy, sigmoidoscopy, colonoscopy, and endoscopic retrograde cholangiopancreatography can all be performed in pregnancy if there are no alternative options. They should be performed by an experienced operator, with the lowest amount of sedation, and ideally in the second trimester. After 20 weeks of gestation, the position of the woman needs to be carefully considered to optimize procedural success and minimize aortocaval compression from the gravid uterus.

3. What treatment would you offer this woman to treat her current symptoms?

Most women with a flare of Crohn's disease can be managed as an outpatient. Treatment of a flare may include 5-aminosalicylic acids or corticosteroids. In Crohn's disease these are mainly oral treatments, but sigmoid or rectal disease may respond to local treatments such as enemas. Women should stop non-steroidal anti-inflammatories as they may worsen bowel symptoms.

Women with more severe disease may require hospital admission. They may require intravenous fluids, intravenous steroids, antibiotics, and nutritional support. Surgery may be needed in the acute setting for the same indications as outside of pregnancy, but this may be a complicated decision particularly in the third trimester. In some women with aggressive disease and a flare in pregnancy, it may be appropriate to start biological therapy in pregnancy.

VTE prophylaxis should be considered in all women with a flare of inflammatory bowel disease.

4. What other treatments can be used to treat inflammatory bowel disease in pregnancy?

The following treatments are safe in pregnancy and breastfeeding:

- 5-aminosalicylic acids (oral and enemas)
- Corticosteroids (oral, intravenous and enemas)
- Sulfasalazine (this interferes with folate absorption so women should be taking 5 mg folic acid daily throughout pregnancy).
- Azathioprine and 6-mercaptopurine
- Ciclosporin
- Tacrolimus
- Anti-TNF therapies

Biological therapies are increasingly used in women of childbearing age. TNF inhibitors are safe throughout pregnancy with no evidence that they cause congenital abnormalities. Stopping TNF inhibitors can risk a disease flare in pregnancy and postpartum, as well as increasing the risk of preterm birth and intrauterine growth restriction. However, the antibody structure of these therapies mean that all except certolizumab cross the placenta in the later stages of pregnancy, and the infant blood level can be the same (or greater in some cases) as that of the mother, which increases the potential for immunosuppression in the neonate. To that end, all women who receive biological therapies should be counselled about the risks and benefits of stopping or continuing these drugs, and decisions made on an individual basis. If the TNF inhibitor therapy is continued in the second half of pregnancy, live vaccine administration to the baby should be avoided in the first 6 months of their life (12 months for infliximab). The live vaccines given in the UK vaccination schedule in the first 6 months are rotavirus and BCG.

There is little evidence about use of vedolizumab, ustekinumab, or tofacitinib in pregnancy. The lack of evidence but also the risk of disease destabilization if the medications are stopped should be discussed with all women on these as part of pre-conception counselling.

Methotrexate, leflunamide, and mycophenolate mofetil are known to be terato-genic and should be avoided in pregnancy and prior to conception.

5. What are the risks associated with inflammatory bowel disease in pregnancy?

Women with quiescent IBD have no increased risk of adverse pregnancy outcomes, for mother or for the fetus. There is no increased risk of congenital abnormalities in women with inflammatory bowel disease if they are on appropriate medication.

Active IBD in pregnancy, particularly in early pregnancy and conception, is associated with fetal risks including low birth weight, small for gestational age babies, and preterm birth, as well as maternal risks such as venous thromboembolism and pre-eclampsia.

One-third of women with IBD experience a flare after pregnancy. Women who are treated with anti-TNF therapies prior to pregnancy and stop their biological therapy during pregnancy are at increased risk of a flare in pregnancy or the postpartum period.

6. What mode of delivery should be recommended for this woman?

Most women with inflammatory bowel disease can have a vaginal birth. However, caesarean delivery may be preferable in some women, particularly those with active perianal or rectal disease, previous perianal disease, an ileo-anal pouch, or ileo-rectal anastomosis. There is a risk that vaginal birth and instrumentation may affect continence or cause a worsening of perianal disease or fistula formation. Dedicated imaging such as MRI scans may be useful to assess the extent of perianal disease in pregnancy.

Mode and timing of birth should be discussed in a multidisciplinary team, and this should include colorectal surgeons, especially in women with active intra-abdominal inflammation or previous intra-abdominal surgery. Mode of birth should nevertheless be predominantly driven by obstetric considerations. The time of birth may be brought forward to allow elective birth rather than emergency surgery in some cases.

Further reading

1. C. Lamb *et al.* British Society of Gastroenterology consensus guidelines on the management of inflammatory bowel disease in adults. Gut. 2019; 68:s1–106.
2. U. Mahadevan *et al.* Inflammatory bowel disease in pregnancy clinical care pathway: A Report from the American Gastroenterological Association IBD Parenthood Project Working Group. Gastroenterology. 2019;156(5):1508–24.

Case 29

A 35-year-old woman was pregnant for the first time. She had no significant past medical history. When she booked with her midwife, she had a normal blood pressure (105/70 mmHg), and a urine sample was sent for culture. No dipstick results were documented. Her BMI was 42 kg/m². At her 16-week antenatal visit she was noted to have 2+ protein on dipstick, which was confirmed by a urinary protein:creatinine ratio of 100 mg/mmol. Her blood pressure remained normal, she had no symptoms of urinary tract infection, and she was entirely well.

Initial assessment

General inspection: Well in herself
Heart rate: 88 bpm
Blood pressure: 100/70 mmHg
Respiratory rate: 16 breaths/minute
Temperature: 36.2 °C
Oxygen saturations: 100% on room air
Urinalysis: 2+ protein, no nitrites

Examination

Cardiovascular: Normal heart sounds, no murmurs
Respiratory: Normal breath sounds
Abdomen: Soft and non-tender. No organomegaly. Gravid uterus appropriate size for dates

Bloods

See Table 29.1.

Table 29.1 Bloods

Haemoglobin	112 g/L
WCC	6.5×10^9/L
Platelets	212×10^9/L
Sodium	136 mmol/L
Potassium	4.0 mmol/L
Urea	1.5 mmol/L
Creatinine	55 µmol/L
Bilirubin	6 µmol/L
ALT	12 iU/L
Albumin	29 g/L

Questions

1. What are the potential causes for the proteinuria?
2. What tests might you arrange?
3. When would you consider a renal biopsy?
4. What monitoring would you arrange?

Answers

1. What are the potential causes for the proteinuria?

Urinary protein can be the result of glomerular or tubular leak, or overflow of pathological circulating proteins such as light chains.

Physiological proteinuria can be seen in association with exercise, infection, or upright posture.

ACE inhibitor discontinuation can lead to a significant increase in proteinuria.

A wide range of *renal disease* can cause proteinuria. Of relevance in this case is obesity-related glomerulopathy, which is increasingly being recognized as a cause of proteinuria that persists beyond pregnancy.

Gestational proteinuria commonly develops in pregnancy, and whilst some women go on to develop pre-eclampsia, this is not guaranteed. It is often quoted that if proteinuria develops after 20 weeks of gestation, it is likely to be gestational proteinuria, but this cut-off is clearly not absolute so women where proteinuria is identified after 20 weeks should still be reviewed with underlying renal disease in mind. In this case, the identification at 16 weeks makes gestational proteinuria less likely, and the absence of a urine protein assessment at the booking visit increases the possibility that the proteinuria was present prior to pregnancy.

2. What tests might you arrange?

Urinary protein:creatinine ratio (PCR) is a spot test that is approximately equivalent to a 24-hour urine collection but is much more achievable in real-world clinical practice. The upper limit of normal in pregnancy is regarded as 30 mg/mmol (approximately equivalent to 300 mg in 24 hr).

Urinary albumin:creatinine ratio (ACR) is a more sensitive test than PCR so may well be increasingly used in the next few years (the upper limit of normal in pregnancy being 8 mg/mmol).

Blood tests to look for both underlying pathology and consequences of increased protein loss, should be performed, and include:

- Renal function
- Albumin
- ANA, ANCA, anti-dsDNA, immunoglobulins, C3/4
- HbA1c if risk factors for T2DM
- Antiphospholipase A2 receptor antibodies

Renal ultrasound is an important initial test to identify any structural abnormalities that may not have previously been clinically apparent.

PLGF-based testing (either PLGF or sFlt-1:PLGF ratio) has recently been introduced into widespread clinical use and is validated for use between 20 and 34 weeks and 6 days of gestation. A reduction in PLGF, or an increase in the ratio, can be seen before pre-eclampsia presents clinically. This may therefore be of use if other features that overlap with that of pre-eclampsia are also present, to aid the distinction between a hypertensive disorder of pregnancy and an underlying renal cause. In this case, she is too early in gestation for this to be used.

3. When would you consider a renal biopsy?

A renal biopsy can be performed in pregnancy, but with increasing gestation comes an increasing risk of bleeding. It should therefore be reserved for clinical situations where the results would lead to a change in management during pregnancy and cannot wait until after birth, for example:

- Heavy proteinuria and nephrotic syndrome
- Suspicion of intrinsic renal disease such as vasculitis where there is no other appropriate site for biopsy
- Suspicion of early-onset pre-eclampsia where the differential is lupus nephritis

It should always be performed by an experienced operator.

4. What monitoring would you arrange?

If all blood tests and imaging are reassuring, it is appropriate to continue to monitor blood pressure and proteinuria throughout pregnancy in case hypertension or and pre-eclampsia develops. This is often performed at a frequency of 2–4 weekly but will depend on local protocols.

It is important to repeat the protein quantification as a significant increase could reflect super-imposed pre-eclampsia, but also because VTE prophylaxis with LMWH is indicated if nephrotic-range proteinuria develops (defined as a PCR of 300 mg/mmol or over, equivalent to 3 g in 24 hr).

She was monitored regularly, and her blood pressure remained normal. At her 28-week visit, proteinuria is again noted, but haematuria is also identified on urinalysis.

Questions

5. What are the possible causes of microscopic (non-visible) haematuria?
6. She does not develop hypertension and has a vaginal birth following the spontaneous onset of labour at 39 weeks of gestation. What follow-up might you arrange?

Answers

5. What are the possible causes of microscopic (non-visible) haematuria?

Microscopic (non-visible) haematuria is a common finding in pregnancy but rarely represents a concerning underlying cause. False positive results on urinalysis can result from myoglobinuria, strenuous exercise, contamination with vaginal secretions or vaginal candidiasis. Even if the presence of red cells is confirmed on microscopy, it is still possible that this is not reflective of pathology and may resolve after birth.

The coexistence of haematuria and proteinuria, however, points more to a pathological cause, and urgent microscopy should be performed to confirm the presence of red cell casts, which in combination with proteinuria, is suggestive of active glomerulonephritis.

6. She does not develop hypertension and has a vaginal birth following the spontaneous onset of labour at 39 weeks of gestation. What follow-up might you arrange after delivery?

Proteinuria identified in pregnancy may well resolve in the weeks following birth. Renal referral is therefore advised if proteinuria persists for over 12 weeks. Effective contraception in the short term is advisable to enable investigation as needed before a further pregnancy is undertaken.

Case 30

A 22-year-old woman was pregnant for the first time. At 36 weeks of gestation she presented with a 3-day history of worsening left-sided lower back pain. She had no gastrointestinal or urinary symptoms, and no symptoms in her legs, for example paraesthesia, numbness, or swelling. Her pregnancy had been uncomplicated prior to this presentation; her booking blood pressure was normal (100/60 mmHg) and her BMI was 24 kg/m². She had no significant past medical history or family history. She took pregnancy multivitamins and no other medications.

Initial assessment

General inspection:	Well, uncomfortable
Heart rate:	98 bpm
Blood pressure:	105/65 mmHg
Respiratory rate:	16 breaths/minute
Temperature:	36.4 °C
Oxygen saturations:	99% on room air
Urinalysis:	No protein

Examination

Cardiovascular:	Normal heart sounds, no murmurs
Respiratory:	Normal breath sounds
Abdomen:	No organomegaly. Gravid uterus appropriate size for dates, soft and non-tender on palpation. No symphysis pubis tenderness
Back:	No tenderness over vertebral spinous processes or sacroiliac joints Tenderness in left flank
Legs:	No swelling

Bloods

See Table 30.1.

Table 30.1 Bloods

Haemoglobin	109 g/L
WCC	9.7×10^9/L
Platelets	154×10^9/L
Sodium	135 mmol/L
Potassium	3.6 mmol/L
Urea	2.1 mmol/L
Creatinine	54 µmol/L
Bilirubin	7 µmol/L
ALT	21 iU/L
Albumin	31 g/L
CRP	38 mg/L
PT	11.2 s
APTT	26.5 s

Questions

1. What are the possible causes for her back pain?
2. What investigations might be useful?

Answers

1. What are the possible causes for her back pain?

Obstetric causes including preterm labour, placental abruption, or uterine rupture are important to consider in any woman presenting with back pain. These would typically be experienced as abdominal pain, with corroborating findings on abdominal palpation. Complications of uterine fibroids or ovarian cysts may also cause back pain.

Pyelonephritis is a common cause of loin pain in pregnancy, but the pain is often associated with urinary symptoms and/or features of infection or sepsis. Whilst urinalysis often shows abnormalities in the setting of urinary tract infection such as the presence of leucocytes, nitrites, or protein, they are not sensitive or specific for infection and a urine culture should always be sent. Urine and blood cultures are important, and a low threshold for starting antibiotic treatment should be used if infection is suspected.

Nephrolithiasis (renal stones) can cause acute, severe loin pain which often occurs in the absence of systemic symptoms or blood test abnormalities. An infected, obstructed kidney is a rare occurrence but is concerning and requires urgent intervention. This should therefore always be considered in women with renal colic or symptoms of pyelonephritis.

Proximal deep venous thrombosis is another possibility, as this can cause pain in the absence of other symptoms such as leg swelling. Whilst venous thromboembolism risk factors are repeatedly assessed at routine antenatal appointments, VTE is still seen in women in the absence of risk factors and cannot be excluded on this basis alone.

Muscular back pain is common in pregnancy but should be viewed as a diagnosis of exclusion unless there is a clear history of lifting or twisting. Pelvic girdle pain (PGP, also known as symphysis pubis dysfunction or SPD) is common, presenting with low pelvic pain anteriorly (symphysis pubis) and posteriorly (sacroiliac joints). Pain is typically worse on mobilizing, particularly rolling over in bed or rising from a chair. The pain can be elicited when palpating over the affected joints. PGP may be associated with sciatica.

Neurological causes such as sciatica are sometimes described as back pain, but typically sciatica will produce sudden, sharp pain in the back that may radiate down one leg.

2. What investigations might be useful?

Specific blood tests include blood cultures and CRP. Whilst D-dimers are used in non-pregnant individuals in the risk stratification for VTE, these are not validated for use in pregnancy and not recommended by RCOG guidelines in the assessment of women with a potential VTE.

Imaging is important and it would be reasonable to arrange ultrasound of abdomen (to include kidneys) and Doppler ultrasonography of the veins of the upper leg, as this is a readily available resource and may identify an abnormality to explain the symptoms. If this does not, then MRI abdomen should be considered.

The patient undergoes ultrasound of her abdomen and legs and no abnormality is identified. Whilst an inpatient she has required opioid analgesia for the pain. An MRI abdomen was therefore performed which identified extensive left-sided iliofemoral DVT.

Questions

3. What treatment options are available?
4. What monitoring is required?
5. What advice do you give about delivery?
6. What impact does this have on future pregnancies?

Answers

3. What treatment options are available?

Therapeutic anticoagulation is mandated in the absence of contra-indications. LMWH is the standard treatment in pregnancy, in once or twice daily dosing, but in some countries unfractionated heparin is used (either multiple doses a day or an intravenous infusion).

Catheter-directed thrombolysis is increasingly being considered as a treatment option for pulmonary emboli or large DVT, but in this individual there is not an indication to perform this, in the absence of severe venous compromise to her left leg.

An inferior vena caval filter is sometimes considered if anticoagulation is contra-indicated or if a procedure is required imminently and anticoagulation cannot be safely administered.

4. What monitoring is required?

Anti-Xa monitoring is advised in the RCOG guidelines for women at extremes of weight (defined as below 50 kg or over 90 kg), have renal impairment, or a history of recurrent VTE whilst on anticoagulation. The target anti-Xa varies slightly depending on the type of LMWH due to differing anti-Xa and IIa activity of the different types of LMWH available but is usually in the range of 0.6–1.0 iU/ml for the treatment of VTE.

Unfractionated heparin is traditionally monitored by using the APTT, but this is particularly unreliable in the third trimester, as the physiological increase in factor VIII leads to a shortened APTT. Apparent heparin resistance may therefore be seen when solely using APTT monitoring at this time in pregnancy, and it is recommended that anti-Xa monitoring is used in preference. The anti-Xa target for unfractionated heparin is 0.3–0.7 iU/ml.

5. What advice do you give her about delivery?

There is no urgent indication for delivery in this case, indeed the greater the time between this event and delivery the better, for clot stabilization. If she labours spontaneously soon, or urgent delivery for other reasons is required, then options include an unfractionated heparin infusion and/or an IVC filter but an MDT discussion is advisable in this setting.

If delivery is more than 2 weeks after the acute VTE, then a short time without anticoagulation is less of a risk to maternal health. Some centres advocate planned induction of labour to enable careful timing of doses, for example the last dose of therapeutic LMWH 24 hours prior to admission for induction so that neuraxial techniques are not contra-indicated.

Anticoagulation treatment after birth should be continued to enable a total of at least 3 months treatment to be completed.

6. What impact does this have on future pregnancies?

The occurrence of oestrogen-related VTE mandates the recommendation of prophylactic LMWH in any future pregnancy, from a positive pregnancy test onwards, throughout pregnancy and until 6 weeks postnatally.

Further reading

1. RCOG: Thrombosis and embolism during pregnancy and the puerperium: Acute management (Green top guideline No 37b, April 2015).<https://www.rcog.org.uk/globalassets/documents/guidelines/gtg-37b.pdf>

Case 31

A 33-year-old woman attended for pre-pregnancy counselling. She had a history of chronic kidney disease having presented at the age of 18 with severe hypertension. She had been found to have bilateral small kidneys on ultrasound and a biopsy had not been performed. She was started on peritoneal dialysis via Tenckhoff catheter at the age of 21 and had a non-related donor transplant at the age of 26. She had remained very well since the transplant with no episodes of rejection. Her maintenance treatment was tacrolimus and azathioprine. She remained normotensive and had no proteinuria.

She was planning a cycle of *in vitro* fertilization because of a history of polycystic ovarian syndrome and anovulation. Previous ovulation induction with letrozole had not been successful.

Her most recent blood tests showed a haemoglobin of 110 g/L, creatinine 100 µmol/L with normal electrolytes and bicarbonate.

Questions

1. How should women with renal transplants be counselled about future pregnancy?
2. What adjustments need to be made to her medication regime in advance of pregnancy?
3. What advice would you give her about undergoing an IVF cycle?
4. Does the presence of a renal transplant influence plans for egg collection during the IVF cycle?
5. What would the ideal management be during a pregnancy?

Answers

1. How should women with renal transplants be counselled about future pregnancy?

Women should usually be advised to delay conception until at least a year of stable renal function following a transplant and use effective contraception in this period. The best outcomes are achieved if pregnancy occurs 1–5 years after transplantation, with normal renal function and no hypertension or proteinuria. Referral to a geneticist is advised if the underlying cause of the renal impairment is genetic, such as polycystic kidney disease.

The increased cardiac output in pregnancy results in an increased glomerular filtration rate. In women with renal transplants, as in women with kidney disease without a transplant, pregnancy can lead to a decline in renal function, particularly in the latter stages of pregnancy. This deterioration may recover after birth, but this is not always the case. There is therefore a chance of a step down in transplant function as a result of pregnancy, particularly in women with a lower GFR prior to pregnancy.

Impaired kidney function, irrespective of the presence of transplant or native kidneys, is associated with a variety of pregnancy complications:

- Hypertensive disorders of pregnancy
- Urinary tract infection
- Preterm birth (spontaneous or iatrogenic)
- Low birthweight babies
- Neonatal mortality
- Venous thromboembolism (if significant proteinuria present)
- Increased risk of operative birth/caesarean delivery
- Hyperglycaemia (related to steroid or tacrolimus use)

The chance of these developing is increased if hypertension and/or proteinuria is present.

Women on immunosuppression have an increased risk of cervical cancer, so it is important to ensure they are attending their regular screening when it is offered.

2. What adjustments need to be made to her medication regime in advance of pregnancy?

Medications such as prednisolone, tacrolimus, and azathioprine can be continued in pregnancy, in contrast to mycophenolate mofetil and sirolimus which should be discontinued in advance of conception and replaced with an appropriate alternative.

Tacrolimus levels need to be monitored carefully from early pregnancy as the physiological changes in pregnancy lead to a reduction in drug level, so a higher dose is usually needed.

Iron, haemoglobin, calcium, and phosphate should all be measured, and any deficiencies replaced with the appropriate supplementation, ideally prior to conception.

Folic acid should be prescribed according to local/national antenatal guidelines.

3. What advice would you give her about undergoing an IVF cycle?

A *fresh cycle* of IVF involves several stages, which include downregulation of pituitary LH and FSH release, ovarian stimulation with synthetic follicle-stimulating hormone, oocyte maturation with a one-off dose of HCG, and then transvaginal ultrasound-guided egg collection carefully timed after the HCG dose. The collected eggs are then combined with sperm to be fertilized and allowed to develop for several days before being replaced. The timing of replacement depends on the quality of the resulting embryos as well as the quantity. If sufficient good quality embryos develop then they will be kept longer to develop to blastocyst stage, as transfer of a blastocyst is associated with higher success rates. However, if very few embryos result, then they may be replaced earlier due to the risk of not surviving until this stage of development.

A *frozen embryo transfer* is when good quality embryos created after egg collection are frozen, which can then be defrosted and replaced later, either into the same person they were collected from, or into a surrogate. A frozen cycle can either be 'natural' or 'medicated'. The former is when the endometrial thickness of the uterus during the woman's menstrual cycle is monitored, and the embryo replaced when the thickness is deemed adequate. The latter is when the endometrial thickness is enhanced with exogenous oestrogen and then maintained with progesterone supplementation, and when ultrasound monitoring deems the thickness to be adequate, the embryo is replaced.

There are risks associated with all IVF cycles:

- Ovarian hyperstimulation syndrome (OHSS) occurs as a result of excessive oestrogen levels from the overstimulated ovaries, which can lead to ascites, effusions, and can be life-threatening if severe
- Venous thromboembolism associated with increased oestrogen (endogenous or exogenous), and OHSS
- Bleeding at the time of egg collection
- Multiple pregnancy because of multiple embryo transfer, or spontaneous twinning from a single embryo
- Pelvic infection related to egg collection

There are no data yet about the risks of IVF in women with renal disease or renal transplants. It is likely, however, that OHSS could be more problematic in women with impaired renal function and therefore theoretically less able to deal with the fluid shifts in this condition. One option to mitigate this potential risk is to do a 'freeze all' cycle following egg collection, which allows the woman time to recover from egg collection and ovarian stimulation, and then after several weeks/months, she can undergo a frozen cycle, without the risk of OHSS.

It is also likely that the risk of infection related to egg collection is increased in women who are immunosuppressed, but this risk has not been quantified and no policy for routine antibiotic prophylaxis exists for this group of women.

Single embryo transfer is increasingly being recommended for the majority, if not all, women undergoing IVF due to the known risks of multiple pregnancy. In women with medical conditions such as renal transplants, these risks are increased further so single embryo transfer is strongly advised.

4. Does the presence of a renal transplant influence plans for egg collection during the IVF cycle?

Potential complication of egg collection in all women include bleeding, infection, and injury to other pelvic structures. It is performed transvaginally, guided by transvaginal ultrasound. It is therefore theoretically possible that damage to surrounding structures such as a kidney transplant located in or near the pelvis could occur, but this has not been reported.

5. What would the ideal management be during a pregnancy?

Women with renal transplants, particularly those with multiple transplants, are best managed in pregnancy by a multidisciplinary team including transplant physicians and surgeons, usually at a transplant centre.

Early and regular assessment of tacrolimus levels are crucial and an increase in dose is required if the level is lower than the target range. Folic acid should also be continued until at least 12 weeks of gestation (or started if not on prior to conception).

Priorities throughout pregnancy include regular review for renal function, drug monitoring, blood pressure and proteinuria assessment, assessment of Hb and treatment of anaemia, regular fetal growth scans, and screening for gestational diabetes (if on tacrolimus or prednisolone or with other risk factors for GDM). Careful prescribing of medications during pregnancy is also required as some commonly used medications can interact with immunosuppressive agents, an example of which is erythromycin and tacrolimus.

If an increase in creatinine occurs, graft rejection must be considered and in some cases a transplant biopsy will be required to clarify this.

There is no medical reason why a caesarean section is required, so this can be reserved for obstetric indications, but it is advisable for obstetricians to familiarize themselves with the previous surgical procedures and resulting anatomical changes prior to a planned delivery.

Further reading

1. **K. Wiles** *et al.* The Renal Association Clinical Practice Guideline pregnancy and renal disease. 2019. <https://ukkidney.org/sites/renal.org/files/FINAL-Pregnancy-Guideline-September-2019.pdf>

2. Intrapartum care for women with existing medical conditions or obstetric complications and their babies (NICE guideline No 121, 2019). <https://www.nice.org.uk/guidance/ng121>

Case 32

A 29-year-old woman presented at 11 weeks of gestation with a lump in her right breast, which she had first noticed when having a shower a week prior to presentation. There were no associated skin changes, pain, nipple discharge, or other lumps. She had never had anything similar before. Her first pregnancy 3 years previously had been uncomplicated, and she had a vaginal birth after the spontaneous onset of labour at term. She had no past medical history. She was taking pregnancy vitamins and had no known allergies. There was a family history of breast carcinoma in her sister and maternal aunt. She had never smoked and did not drink alcohol.

Initial assessment

General inspection:	Well
Heart rate:	90 bpm
Blood pressure:	95/70 mmHg
Respiratory rate:	12 breaths/min
Temperature:	36.5 °C
Oxygen saturations:	100% on air
Urinalysis:	No protein

Examination

Cardiovascular:	Normal heart sounds, no murmurs
Respiratory:	Reduced breath sounds bilaterally
Abdomen:	Soft abdomen, non-tender gravid uterus
Right breast:	Hard, non-tender, immobile lump, 2 × 2 cm with irregular edges in right upper outer quadrant. Associated axillary lymphadenopathy
Left breast:	Normal

Bloods

See Table 32.1.

Table 32.1 Bloods

Haemoglobin	95 g/L
WCC	8.2 × 10⁹/L
Platelets	550 × 10⁹/L
Sodium	135 mmol/L
Potassium	4.3 mmol/L
Urea	2.9 mmol/L
Creatinine	35 μmol/L
Bilirubin	4 μmol/L
ALT	7 iU/L
ALP	60 iU/L
Albumin	25 g/L
CRP	15 mg/L

Questions

1. What are the possible causes for this breast lump?
2. What are the risk factors for the development of breast cancer?
3. Which investigations are indicated if breast cancer is suspected?
4. What are the management options for this woman in pregnancy?

Answers

1. What are the possible causes for this breast lump?

Breast changes in pregnancy are wide-ranging, and many benign lumps can occur in pregnancy as they can in non-pregnant individuals, such as cysts, fibroadenomas, and fat necrosis. Breast cancer is obviously a possibility, and therefore all women with a breast lump should be referred through the standard pathway for assessment.

2. What are the risk factors for the development of breast cancer?

Breast cancer is the most common malignancy in women, and it is one of the commonest malignancies diagnosed in or soon after pregnancy. Risk factors include:

- Increasing age
- Oestrogen exposure (either endogenous or exogenous), due to a variety of factors including early menarche, nulliparity, late menopause, combined oral contraceptive use, hormone replacement therapy, and increasing age at first full-term pregnancy
- A history of breast cancer on one side increases the risk of developing cancer in the contralateral breast
- Affected first-degree relatives, and the risk increases with the number of first-degree relatives affected, as well as the age at diagnosis
- Genetic mutations include *BRCA1*, *BRCA2*, *p53*, *STK11*, *CDH1*, and *PTEN* are rare, and are seen in approximately 5% of affected women
- Increased alcohol intake
- Smoking

Protective factors:

- Mastectomy (e.g. in those with a known *BRCA1/2* mutation)
- Breastfeeding
- A low-fat diet, particularly in post-menopausal women.

3. What investigations are indicated if breast cancer is suspected?

The assessment pathway in this patient should be the same as in non-pregnant individuals, i.e. urgent referral to a one-stop clinic for clinical review, imaging such as ultrasound (or mammography), and consideration of fine needle aspiration to enable a tissue diagnosis.

If there are concerns around metastatic spread, for example a large or high-grade lesion, lymphadenopathy, or abnormal liver function tests, then a chest radiograph and abdominal ultrasound can be performed. Cross-sectional imaging with CT chest, PET MRI, and ultrasound or radioisotope-guided axillary lymph node biopsy is not contraindicated in pregnancy. Bone scanning and pelvic radiography are not recommended routinely in pregnant women to look for metastases. Plain radiography of bones can be performed if there is a specific concern about localized symptoms that might represent bone metastasis.

This woman has a family history of breast cancer and should be offered genetic counselling and testing for specific breast and breast and ovarian carcinoma syndromes, but the results of this take a long time and are unlikely to make a difference to the decision-making required in a pregnancy.

4. What are the management options for this woman in pregnancy?

Women should be treated as in the non-pregnant population, with some modifications to protect the fetus. Management will depend on the extent, histology, and receptor status of the disease. An MDT approach is important, involving obstetricians, obstetric physicians, breast surgeons, oncologists, midwives, and cancer nurse specialists.

If histology confirms a diagnosis of cancer then an important discussion to have at an early stage is whether to continue the pregnancy. Depending on the gestation of diagnosis, some women in the first or early second trimesters may want to pursue the option of termination of pregnancy followed by treatment of the malignancy. Others may wish to continue the pregnancy and undergo treatment while pregnant, a path chosen by many pregnant women in recent years. This complex decision requires an individualized approach, taking into consideration the woman's personal circumstances (maternal age, existing family, time taken to conceive, desire for future fertility), prognosis of the cancer, and whether pregnancy may impair optimal treatment.

Depending on the type and size of the primary tumour, the normal treatment would be surgery in the first instance (options include mastectomy or wide local excision with or without lymph node clearance). In some cases, neo-adjuvant chemotherapy is advised prior to primary surgery. Wide local excision, mastectomy, breast-conserving surgery, and lymph node dissection can be performed in pregnancy. The potential operating time (surrogate marker for duration of general anaesthesia), the complexity of the procedure and whether it will affect prognosis are important considerations before surgery is undertaken in pregnancy. Sentinel node assessment with radioisotope scintigraphy can be performed in pregnancy as the tracer is mainly taken up in the lymph node. The effect of blue dye tracers on the fetus is unknown so it is recommended that their use is avoided.

Chemotherapy is either given as adjuvant (post-operative systemic medical treatment) or neoadjuvant therapy (use of these agents prior to surgery to induce tumour response).

Chemotherapy is usually avoided in the first trimester due to the potential increase in risk of congenital malformations. Use in the second and third trimesters is not associated with a risk of congenital malformations but there is an increased risk of intrauterine growth restriction, prematurity, and low birth weight. There is, however, the risk that in some women, delaying chemotherapy may affect its efficacy in terms of prognosis.

Anthracyclines are the first-choice chemotherapeutic agent for breast cancer and can be used in pregnancy. Cyclophosphamide and taxanes can also be used if indicated, for example the latter in node-positive disease. Whilst there appears to be minimal risk to the fetus and neonate in the short term, little is known about long-term implications for the child in terms of cardiotoxicity and fertility.

Hormonal therapies such as tamoxifen should be avoided in pregnancy due to the risk of fetal malformations.

HER-2 targeted therapies which include monoclonal antibodies such as pertuzumab and trastuzumab should be avoided in pregnancy due to the risk of fetal renal damage and oligo-anhydramnios. There is little data about small molecule anti-*HER 2* tyrosine kinase inhibitors such as lapatinib in pregnancy. Small molecules, however, can easily cross the placenta so their use is generally avoided in pregnancy.

Radiotherapy should ideally be avoided in pregnancy and delayed until after birth, as the radiation dose to the fetus is greater than that used in imaging. The typical radiation doses used in breast cancer are 46–60 Gy, and the biological absorbed dose of the fetus varies from 0.04 to 2 Gy, with higher exposure in later pregnancy. Depending on the radiotherapy dose and gestation at which this is given, the risks include miscarriage or stillbirth, congenital malformations, impaired growth or development, mutagenic effects, and risk of childhood cancer, but the exact thresholds that these complications occur is not clear.

If radiotherapy is required for life-threatening complications, such as spinal cord compression, then it can be used with fetal shielding and optimization of choice of beam and field.

Immunotherapy using antibodies against programmed cell death protein 1 (PD-1) and the associated ligand (PD-L1) are increasingly being used in the treatment of breast cancer. Inhibition of the PD-1/PD-L1 pathway may cause an immune response against the fetus, as the pathway is involved in the immune tolerance that the mother develops towards the fetus in pregnancy. There is little data of these agents in pregnancy, but in animals they are associated with adverse pregnancy outcomes, so should be avoided at present in pregnancy.

Other important considerations in pregnant women with active malignancy include:

- VTE prophylaxis
- Antiemetics
- Proton pump inhibitor
- G-CSF can be used if required for leukopenia

Delivery mode and timing depend on her treatment plans and fetal assessment with regular growth scans. If chemotherapy is initiated in pregnancy following surgery, then the ideal scenario is that birth is planned for term, allowing an interval between chemotherapy cycle and birth to enable bone marrow recovery prior to birth and therefore reduce the risks of bleeding and sepsis at that time. A caesarean delivery is not mandated by the diagnosis of cancer in pregnancy, and particularly as she has had a previous uncomplicated vaginal birth, it would be appropriate to aim for an induction of labour.

Breastfeeding after birth depends on treatment plans and is usually contraindicated when chemotherapy is restarted, or biological treatment is initiated. There is no evidence that lactation increases the risk of recurrence and a short period of lactation between birth and treatment restarting may be very beneficial to the mother from a psychological perspective. The relatively recent development of donor milk banks help infants born to women having chemotherapy to continue receiving breast milk even if it is not possible to use their mother's own.

Postnatal contraception is important to discuss, and non-hormonal methods should be advised. The copper intrauterine device is therefore the most reliable option. Preventing further pregnancy until treatment is completed allows for optimal treatment choices.

She undergoes right mastectomy and axillary lymph node clearance. A diagnosis of oestrogen and progesterone receptor positive breast cancer is made with 10 out of 25 nodes positive. A plan is made for chemotherapy to start 6 weeks after surgery: 4 cycles of EC chemotherapy (every 3 weeks) followed by weekly paclitaxel. She starts this at 21 weeks of gestation and her first three cycles are uneventful. A few days after her fourth cycle however, at 31 weeks of gestation, she presents to the labour ward with a fever and feeling unwell.

Initial assessment

General inspection: Unwell, vasodilated, septic
Heart rate: 130 bpm
Blood pressure: 70/50 mmHg
Respiratory rate: 25 breaths/min
Temperature: 38.9 °C
Oxygen saturations: 97% on air
Urinalysis: No protein

Bloods

See Table 32.2.

Table 32.2 Repeat bloods

Haemoglobin	80 g/L
WCC	1.2×10^9/L
Neutrophils	0.1×10^9/L
Platelets	110×10^9/L
CRP	70 mg/L

Questions

5. What is the diagnosis?
6. How would you treat her?

Answers

5. What is the diagnosis?

This woman has signs consistent with neutropenic sepsis, as defined by NICE as fever of 38 °C or higher, or symptoms and signs of sepsis, in a person receiving chemotherapy with a neutrophil count of less than 0.5×10^9/L. It is a medical emergency and maternal sepsis is associated with significant maternal and fetal morbidity.

6. How would you treat her?

Urgent investigations should include bloods (FBC, renal function, liver function, CRP, lactate), blood cultures, urine culture, cultures of any wounds or vascular access catheters and chest radiography.

Broad-spectrum antibiotics should be administered, guided by local policies, but usually include antibiotics such as piperacillin and tazobactam, alongside gentamicin.

Fluid resuscitation and careful fluid balance are essential, alongside oxygen if indicated.

G-CSF should be considered.

Fetal assessment should be undertaken but emergency delivery in an unstable mother risks morbidity to both mother and baby, so decisions about birth should be taken by senior obstetricians in conjunction with a multidisciplinary team, which may include physicians in infectious diseases, obstetric medicine, oncology and/or intensive care, obstetricians, and obstetric anaesthetists.

Blood product support depends on her clinical condition and if urgent birth is deemed necessary.

Further reading

1. **L. Benoit** *et al.* Cancer during Pregnancy: A review of pre-clinical and clinical transplacental transfer of anticancer agents. Cancers. 2021; **13**(6): 1238.
2. **F. Poggio** *et al.* Update on the management of breast cancer during pregnancy. Cancers. 2020; **12** (12): 3616.
3. RCOG: Pregnancy and breast cancer (Green top Guideline No 12, 2011). <https://www.rcog.org.uk/en/guidelines-research-services/guidelines/gtg12/>

Case 33

A 20-year-old woman in her first pregnancy presented at 29 weeks of gestation with repeated generalized tonic-clonic seizures, without recovery in between. She had been unwell in the preceding 24 hours with vomiting and significantly reduced oral intake. In childhood she had been diagnosed with juvenile myoclonic epilepsy, for which she had been on 75 mg lamotrigine twice daily prior to pregnancy. This dose had not been increased during pregnancy. Prior to this she had had no seizures for over a year. She had no other past medical history and was not taking any other medications. There was no family history of significant illnesses. She had never smoked.

Initial assessment

General inspection:	Unwell, drowsy, post ictal
Heart rate:	120 bpm
Blood pressure:	95/60 mmHg
Respiratory rate:	15 breaths/min
Temperature:	36.8 °C
Oxygen saturations:	100% on 15 L/min oxygen via non-rebreathe mask
Urinalysis:	No protein
Capillary glucose:	5.4 mmol/L

Examination

Cardiovascular:	Normal heart sounds, no murmurs
Respiratory:	Normal breath sounds
Abdomen:	Soft abdomen, non-tender gravid uterus
Neurology:	GCS 3, plantars downgoing, pupils equal and reactive to light

Bloods

See Table 33.1.

Table 33.1 Bloods

Haemoglobin	135 g/L
WCC	8.2×10^9/L
Platelets	150×10^9/L
Sodium	135 mmol/L
Potassium	4.2 mmol/L
Urea	3.1 mmol/L
Creatinine	43 µmol/L
Bilirubin	4 µmol/L
ALT	10 iU/L
ALP	100 iU/L
Albumin	30 g/L
CRP	20 mg/L

Questions

1. What is the explanation for her current clinical condition?
2. What are the possible precipitants for this?
3. How would you treat her in the acute setting?
4. What other investigations would you consider?
5. How would you counsel her about the use of anti-epileptic medication in pregnancy?
6. What are the important considerations in this patient after delivery?

Answers

1. What is the explanation for her current clinical condition?

This woman has status epilepticus, which is a life-threatening condition. It is defined as 5 or more minutes of either continuous seizure activity or repetitive seizures with no intervening recovery of consciousness.

Epilepsy is one of the most common medical conditions in women of child-bearing age. It also remains a significant cause of maternal mortality, mainly because of 'sudden unexpected death in epilepsy' (SUDEP). Seizures in pregnancy can occur for a variety of reasons other than primary epilepsy, including eclampsia, electrolyte abnormalities (such as hypoglycaemia, hypocalcaemia, hyponatraemia), intracranial pathologies (such as cerebral venous sinus thrombosis, intracranial haemorrhage, space-occupying lesion), and infection.

Effective control of seizures is vital as uncontrolled seizures can lead to oxygen deprivation of the fetus secondary to placental hypoperfusion.

In this case there are no other signs to support a diagnosis of eclampsia, and no other reversible causes identified on initial testing.

2. What are the possible precipitants of this?

There are a variety of causes of worsening seizure frequency in pregnancy.

- Poor compliance with medications, often resulting from concerns about the safety of medications in pregnancy.
- Vomiting with reduced absorption of antiepileptic medication.
- Altered pharmacokinetics of drugs in pregnancy, which can result in reduced circulating concentrations of anti-epileptic drugs, particularly lamotrigine.
- Interactions with co-prescribed medications such as antibiotics.
- Sleep deprivation.
- Electrolyte imbalance.

3. How would you treat her in an acute setting?

Status epilepticus is a medical emergency, and requires prompt multidisciplinary management, with involvement of anaesthetist, intensivists, obstetricians, obstetric physicians, and neonatologists.

An 'ABCDE' approach should be undertaken, and any abnormalities identified in this primary survey should be corrected, including abnormal blood glucose. This woman is 29 weeks pregnant, and so should be positioned on her side or with a left lateral tilt.

First-line management of status epilepticus is a benzodiazepine, either intravenously or rectally. If the seizure is ongoing, the dose can be repeated after 10 minutes. If benzodiazepines fail to terminate the seizures, an intravenous infusion of either phenytoin or levetiracetam should then be commenced, the latter being more commonly used in recent years.

Fetal monitoring appropriate for gestation should be undertaken when the mother is stabilized. If there is no evidence of fetal compromise or eclampsia, then delivery is not indicated but this should be reviewed on a very regular basis. Benzodiazepine administration can cause reduced variability in the CTG which usually improves as the benzodiazepine is metabolized and excreted. Decisions about delivery based on CTG monitoring in women who have received benzodiazepines should therefore be discussed at senior level.

If the seizures persist, then sedation with a general anaesthetic, intubation and ventilation is required.

4. What other investigations would you consider?

Drug levels vary widely in pregnancy but should be performed to ensure adequate serum levels. Levels can often fall in pregnancy, secondary to altered drug metabolism, often necessitating a dose increase.

Urinary toxicology to look for evidence of other substances that may have contributed to the seizures.

CT or MRI head is useful if the cause of the increased seizure frequency is not clear from the history, examination, or investigation findings.

Lumbar puncture should be considered if there is any suggestion of intracranial infection.

An electroencephalogram (EEG) is not mandated in a patient who is clearly having epileptiform seizures, however if there is doubt about the diagnosis (e.g. if non-epileptiform seizures are a possibility) then this is a useful test.

5. How would you counsel her about the use of anti-epileptic medication in pregnancy?

Seizure control is essential in pregnancy to minimize risks to the fetus and the mother. Women with epilepsy are more likely to have babies who are small for gestational age or delivered preterm, and frequent seizures in pregnancy are associated with developmental delay in the neonate.

Many anti-epileptic drugs are associated with teratogenicity when used in the first trimester, and this varies with the type and dose of drug, as well as the number of drugs being taken. Epilepsy should therefore ideally be controlled with the lowest dose possible and with the fewest number of medications. Common malformations include neural tube defects, cardiac abnormalities, facial clefts, and genitourinary abnormalities, as well as developmental delay. Women on anticonvulsants are recommended to take high-dose folic acid for at least 3 months prior to conception and during the first 12 weeks of pregnancy to reduce the risk of neural tube defects.

Lamotrigine and levetiracetam are the preferred agents for use in pregnancy as they do not increase the risk of congenital abnormalities. Carbamazepine is also commonly used but increases the rate of congenital abnormalities from a background rate of 2–3% to approximately 4–5%. If valproate is used, the rate of malformation is between 10% and 25%, as well as increasing the risk of developmental delay. This is unacceptably high and has led to the Medicines and Healthcare product Regulatory Agency (MHRA) in the United Kingdom issuing a recent update that clearly states 'valproate medicines must no longer be used in women or girls of childbearing potential unless a Pregnancy Prevention Programme is in place'. In most cases, treatment with multiple anticonvulsants increases the risk of malformations further than any individual drug. Clobazam is appropriate to use in pregnancy and is often used to bridge dose adjustments or new medications as well as in labour if there is a concern that seizures may increase in frequency.

It should be noted that levels of lamotrigine and, to a lesser extent, levetiracetam can fall dramatically during pregnancy, often necessitating significant dose increases. There are no guidelines about the frequency or utility of measuring anticonvulsant drug levels during pregnancy, but there is some evidence that ensuring drug levels are in the therapeutic range can reduce seizure frequency. Drug level monitoring can also be useful in women where there is an increase in seizure frequency, a change in dose, or if there are concerns about drug compliance. Any dose changes should be reviewed postpartum with a planned reduction to pre-pregnancy doses in the first few weeks after birth.

6. What are the important considerations in this patient after delivery?

Drug doses should be reviewed, and it is likely that a planned reduction to pre-pregnancy doses in the first few weeks after delivery will be required.

Postnatal contraception should be discussed to minimize the risk of an unplanned pregnancy. Several anti-epileptic drugs, such as phenytoin and carbamazepine, are hepatic enzyme inducers, thus reducing the efficacy of the combined oral contraceptive or the progesterone-only pill. Oestrogen can induce the metabolism of lamotrigine and therefore may lower drug levels, so alternatives to the combined oral contraceptive is often preferred in women on this. Both hormonal and non-hormonal coils as well as methoxyprogesterone injections are effective and typically safe for all anticonvulsant medications.

Safety precautions when caring for a new baby should also be discussed, due to the increased risk of seizures in the postpartum period, due to sleep deprivation and other triggers specific to each patient. Examples of this include changing the baby's nappy on the floor (as opposed to at a height on a changing table), bathing the baby in shallow water when other adults are in the house, and avoidance of co-sleeping.

Further reading

1. RCOG: Epilepsy in pregnancy (Green-top Guideline No 68). <https://www.rcog.org.uk/en/gui delines-research-services/guidelines/gtg68/>

2. Medicines & Healthcare Products Regulatory Agency. Antiepileptic drugs: Review of safety of use during pregnancy (2021). <https://www.gov.uk/government/publications/public-assesm ent-report-of-antiepileptic-drugs-review-of-safety-of-use-during-pregnancy/antiepileptic-drugs-review-of-safety-of-use-during-pregnancy>

3. NICE pathway and clinical knowledge summary: Epilepsy <https://cks.nice.org.uk/topics/epilepsy/>

Case 34

A 38-year-old woman was brought to the Emergency Department at 28 weeks of gestation. She was unwell, complaining of acute severe epigastric pain and vomiting for the preceding 8 hours. She complained of mild constipation throughout pregnancy, but last opened her bowels 2 days previously. She had no fever and no other symptoms.

The pregnancy was uneventful aside from nausea and vomiting in the first trimester. This was her second pregnancy, her first being 10 years previously. She was diagnosed with gestational diabetes in that pregnancy. Two years prior to this pregnancy she underwent a Roux-en-Y gastric bypass. Her BMI at the start of pregnancy was 26 kg/m², having been 39 kg/m² prior to surgery.

Initial assessment

General inspection:	GCS 15/15 but unable to complete talk in full sentences due to pain
Heart rate:	100 beats per minute, regular
Blood pressure:	105/55 mmHg
Respiratory rate:	28 breaths per minute
Oxygen saturations:	98% on room air
Temperature:	36.9 °C
Urinalysis:	Glucose 3+

Examination

Cardiovascular:	Normal heart sounds, no added sounds
Respiratory:	Normal breath sounds throughout
Abdomen:	Tender in the right hypochondrium with guarding; tinkling bowel sounds

Bloods

See Table 34.1.

Table 34.1 Bloods

Haemoglobin	121 g/L
WCC	10.3 × 10⁹/L
Platelets	273 × 10⁹/L
Sodium	138 mmol/L
Potassium	4.2 mmol/L
Urea	5 mmol/L
Creatinine	55 μmol/L
Bilirubin	18 μmol/L
ALT	11 iU/L
ALP	68 iU/L
Albumin	37 g/L
CRP	6 mg/L

Questions

1. What are the potential causes for this presentation?
2. What investigations would you arrange?
3. What treatment would you give her?
4. What nutritional and vitamin supplements are recommended for women who are pregnant and previously underwent bariatric surgery?
5. How do you test for gestational diabetes in a woman who has undergone bariatric surgery?

Answers

1. What are the potential causes for this presentation?

Severe abdominal pain and new-onset vomiting after the first trimester should always raise the possibility of an underlying surgical complication, particularly in a woman with previous bariatric surgery.

Internal herniation causing small bowel obstruction is a complication of gastric bypass and is more common in pregnancy than in non-pregnant individuals, with a reported incidence of up to 8%. It is most often seen after laparoscopic procedures rather than open surgery. Abdominal pain is always present, and nausea and vomiting are seen in 50% of cases. This is an emergency, associated with maternal and fetal mortality (9% and 13% respectively).

Acute pancreatitis is a rare but severe disease in pregnancy. The most common causes are gallstones, alcohol excess, and familial hypertriglyceridaemia, but in many cases a specific cause is never identified. It is more common in the third trimester, causing abdominal pain, nausea, vomiting, anorexia, and fever. The risks of acute pancreatitis in pregnancy include preterm labour and stillbirth.

Biliary tract disease and gallstones are common in women of childbearing age. Up to 30% of pregnancies are complicated by gallbladder sludge, and up to 12% of pregnant women have gallstones. Biliary disease is more common in the third trimester due to the increased oestrogen levels. However, biliary colic, acute cholecystitis, and acute cholangitis are rare in pregnancy. Nevertheless, these are associated with preterm birth and stillbirth.

Appendicitis is the most common non-obstetric surgical condition in pregnancy, and is most common in the second trimester, though there is an increased risk of appendiceal rupture in the third trimester. Due to the gravid uterus, the pain may not be in the classic location.

Peptic ulceration can occur in pregnancy but is uncommon. In addition to simple peptic ulceration, in a patient with a Roux-en-Y gastric bypass, there is the risk of marginal ulceration along the suture lines. Perforation is a rare but severe complication.

2. What investigations would you arrange?

Additional *blood tests* should include amylase, serum lipase, calcium, and coagulation.

Imaging is also required. In all patients presenting with acute abdominal pain, an erect chest radiograph should be taken to look for air under the diaphragm, which would be consistent with intestinal perforation. A plain abdominal radiograph is often avoided in pregnancy but could be considered as it is easy to obtain and has relatively low radiation exposure and may help by showing evidence of bowel wall thickening consistent with inflammation, or bowel obstruction.

Other imaging modalities include ultrasound, CT and MRI which can all be used for the diagnosis of intra-abdominal sepsis. Ultrasound can be useful to look at biliary disease as well as the kidneys. However, CT or MRI is often required to look with more detail and at other structures. In many surgical cases, such as bowel obstruction from an internal hernia, maternal and fetal outcomes are worse if surgery is delayed. MRI is preferred to CT for abdominal imaging due to the fetal dose of radiation associated with a CT, however if this choice is likely to result in a significant delay in diagnosis and treatment, a CT should be considered.

Additional tests that may be required depending on the clinical scenario include endoscopy, magnetic resonance cholangiopancreatography (MRCP) and endoscopic retrograde cholangiopancreatography (ERCP). All of these can be performed in pregnancy if required but should be performed by an experienced practitioner to ensure appropriate positioning of the pregnant woman and reduction of the time and associated risks of the procedure.

3. What treatment would you give her?

Acute appendicitis and bowel obstruction due to an internal hernia require urgent surgical intervention at any stage in pregnancy. Intravenous fluids, antibiotics, and analgesia will also be required.

Most biliary pathology can be managed conservatively in pregnancy with intravenous fluids, antibiotics, and pain relief. An ERCP may help remove an obstructing stone. In some cases, surgery is warranted, particularly if there is gallbladder perforation or necrosis, or if the woman deteriorates despite conservative management. Cholecystectomy should ideally occur in the second trimester.

Conservative management is often sufficient for pancreatitis, with fluids, nutritional support, antibiotics, and pain relief. ERCP or surgery may be needed if there is a gallstone causing obstructive pancreatitis which does not settle with conservative management. In pancreatitis caused by hypertriglyceridaemia, a very low-fat diet is the first-line treatment. Fixed rate insulin infusions and heparin can also be used to lower triglyceride level. If hypertriglyceridaemia persists, plasma exchange can be used to reduce triglyceride levels.

VTE prophylaxis should be reviewed in all pregnant women admitted with a surgical problem and prescribed as appropriate depending on the clinical situation and timing of potential surgical intervention.

4. What nutritional and vitamin supplements are recommended for women who are pregnant and previously underwent bariatric surgery?

People are at increased risk of micronutrient deficiencies after bariatric surgery. To avoid this, a multivitamin and mineral supplement should be taken daily before conception. A multivitamin should also be used in pregnancy; advice should be sought from a dietician with expertise in bariatric surgery to ensure appropriate supplementation of all micronutrients, especially if a standard pregnancy multivitamin is used. Pregnant women should avoid the retinol form of vitamin A due to the risk of teratogenicity and clinicians should check that the multivitamin contains vitamin A in the beta-carotene form, to avoid overall vitamin A deficiency.

Folic acid supplementation with 5 mg daily is recommended until 12 weeks of gestation. Vitamin D levels should be checked at the start of pregnancy and supplementation should be prescribed in pregnancy and breastfeeding in accordance with local guidelines. Vitamin B12 injections are safe to use in pregnancy and should be used to maintain adequate vitamin B12 levels. Thiamine should be prescribed if there is prolonged vomiting or any malnutrition.

Women who become pregnant following bariatric surgery should have nutritional screening every trimester, including ferritin, folate, vitamin B12, fat-soluble vitamins, and calcium, with additional supplementation as required.

5. How do you test for gestational diabetes in a woman who has undergone bariatric surgery?

All women with a history of bariatric surgery should have their HbA1c and fasting plasma glucose checked at the start of pregnancy to look for pre-existing diabetes.

During pregnancy, an oral glucose tolerance test should not be used to screen for gestational diabetes after bariatric surgery, particularly gastric bypass surgery, due to concerns about accuracy and the risk of dumping syndrome. There is no consensus, however, about the most appropriate way to screen for gestational diabetes after bariatric surgery. Potential screening methods include home blood glucose monitoring (readings 4 times per day for 1–2 weeks between 24 and 28 weeks of gestation), continuous glucose monitoring or 7-point capillary blood glucose profile. Once diagnosed, the same targets for capillary blood glucose should be used as for other pregnant women with gestational diabetes.

Further reading

1. **J. Shawe** *et al.* Pregnancy after bariatric surgery: Consensus recommendations for periconception, antenatal and postnatal care. Obesity Review. 2019; **20**(11): 1507–22.

2. **K. Brown** *et al.* Gallbladder and biliary disease in pregnancy. Clinical Obstetrics and Gynaecology. 2020; **63**(1): 211–25.

3. **G. Ducarme** *et al.* Acute pancreatitis during pregnancy: A review. Journal of Perinatology. 2014; **34**: 87–94.

4. **M. O'Kane** *et al.* British Obesity and Metabolic Surgery Society Guidelines on perioperative and postoperative biochemical monitoring and micronutrient replacement for patients undergoing bariatric surgery—2020 update. Obesity Reviews. 2020; **21**(11): e13087.

Case 35

A 32-year-old woman was brought into the Emergency Department at 32 weeks of gestation. She was unwell and described severe left-sided chest pain and shortness of breath. The pain had started quite suddenly about an hour previously. It was severe, worse on inspiration, and on coughing she could feel the pain radiate to her back. She had noticed some mild right leg swelling and discomfort over the preceding 2 days but had otherwise been well.

This was her first pregnancy and it has been uneventful until this point. She had no significant past medical history and was only taking pregnancy vitamins regularly. Her family history was notable for a pulmonary embolism in her mother after a hip replacement. She worked as a secondary school teacher, lived with her husband, and did not smoke.

Initial assessment

General inspection: GCS 15/15; unable to complete talk in full sentences.
Heart rate: 120 beats per minute, regular
Blood pressure: 90/55 mmHg
Respiratory rate: 28 breaths/min
Oxygen saturation: 95% on 15 L/min oxygen via non-rebreathe mask
Temperature: 36.9 °C
Urinalysis: No protein

Examination

Cardiovascular: Normal heart sounds, no added sounds
Respiratory: Normal breath sounds throughout, no chest tenderness on palpation
Abdomen: Soft, non-tender abdomen, gravid uterus (size appropriate for gestational age)

Bloods

See Table 35.1.

Table 35.1 Bloods

Haemoglobin	121 g/L
WCC	15.3 × 10⁹/L
Platelets	273 × 10⁹/L
Sodium	138 mmol/L
Potassium	4.2 mmol/L
Urea	2.3 mmol/L
Creatinine	53 µmol/L
Bilirubin	7 µmol/L
ALT	14 iU/L
Albumin	30 g/L
CRP	35 mg/L
PT	12.2 s
APTT	26.4 s

Questions

1. What are the important diagnoses to consider in this case?
2. What investigations would you arrange?
3. What treatment would you give her?
4. What effect does a pulmonary embolism have on the mode of delivery?
5. What implication does this have for future pregnancies?

Answers

1. What are the important diagnoses to consider in this case?

Pulmonary embolism is the most common cause for this presentation. Pregnant women are at increased risk of venous thromboembolism due to increased production of clotting factors as well as increased venous stasis due to the gravid uterus. The typical symptoms of pulmonary emboli are the same as those in non-pregnant individuals: shortness of breath, pleuritic chest pain, haemoptysis, pre-syncope, and syncope. Pulmonary embolism can cause acute circulatory collapse and may cause cardiac arrest. Physical examination findings can include tachycardia, hypotension, and hypoxia. A pleural rub may occasionally be heard.

Scoring systems such as the Modified Well's Score are of use in non-pregnant individuals but are not validated for use in pregnancy.

Pleuritis from other causes such as pneumonia or SLE can cause similar symptoms.

Pneumothorax can occur spontaneously ('primary' pneumothorax) or as the result of underlying lung pathology ('secondary'). This diagnosis can be evident from clinical examination (e.g. reduced breath sounds on one side, hyper-resonance, reduced chest expansion on the affected side, subcutaneous emphysema). Any signs of tension pneumothorax such as hypotension and hypoxia mean urgent intervention is required (needle decompression).

Pericarditis can cause chest pain, typically worse on lying down and relieved sitting forwards. This can be idiopathic, related to viral infection or an underlying condition such as SLE. An ECG can show PR depression and saddle ST changes. Assessment of troponin is important to see if there is also myocardial involvement i.e. myopericarditis, which is associated with an increased risk of arrhythmia.

Aortic dissection, although rare, is more common in pregnant individuals compared to non-pregnant individuals, particularly when other medical conditions are present, such as Marfan syndrome or bicuspid aortic valve. It typically presents with a history of chest pain, sometimes with a 'tearing' sensation, that can go to the back (see Case 1) and can result in cardiovascular collapse.

Ischaemic heart disease is becoming more common in pregnancy as women are becoming pregnant later in life. Acute myocardial infarction occurs three times more often in pregnant women than non-pregnant women of a similar age and can cause acute circulatory collapse and cardiac arrest. In less severe cases, atypical symptoms may be misinterpreted as gastro-oesophageal reflux.

Sepsis remains a leading cause of maternal mortality. The common sources of sepsis in pregnancy are urinary tract infection and chorioamnionitis, though all sources of sepsis should be considered. Group A streptococcus is a particular concern in pregnancy (see Case 37). Typical signs of sepsis include pyrexia or hypothermia, tachycardia, tachypnoea, hypoxia, hypotension, oliguria, and impaired consciousness. However pregnant women can show physiological compensation until sepsis is severe. Clinical observations should be charted using the obstetric-specific early warning scores.

2. What investigations would you arrange?

Blood tests should be performed urgently, including FBC, renal function, liver function, coagulation screen, troponin, and BNP. Importantly, there is no merit in checking a D-dimer level as this is of no diagnostic utility in pregnancy.

Arterial blood gas analysis is an important early investigation as this is useful additional information about gas exchange but may also show abnormalities that can contribute to breathlessness (e.g. acidosis).

An ECG may show no abnormalities in pulmonary embolism, but changes including a sinus tachycardia, S1Q3T3 pattern, p pulmonale, right axis deviation, and/or right bundle branch block should all prompt consideration of the diagnosis. However, many of these changes can be seen in normal pregnancy (sinus tachycardia, small Q waves and T wave inversion inferiorly) so these findings may be of limited diagnostic use. An ECG will also help identify arrhythmias and ischaemic changes.

Echocardiography can demonstrate right heart strain, suggestive of pulmonary emboli, as well as other pathology such as valve abnormalities or regional wall motional abnormalities. In an emergency, a bedside echodiogram can be invaluable in identifying or excluding important pathology. A normal echocardiogram, however, does not exclude the diagnosis.

A chest radiograph should be performed in all pregnant women with chest pain or respiratory symptoms.

Computerized tomography pulmonary angiography (CTPA) or ventilation/perfusion scan will confirm the diagnosis of pulmonary embolic disease. If a patient is too unstable to be transferred for urgent imaging, a diagnostic decision needs to be made using other modalities such as echocardiography.

In the non-emergency setting, the recommended first-line investigation is a Doppler ultrasound of the lower limb veins as she has symptoms and signs that might indicate DVT. If a deep vein thrombosis is identified, then a diagnosis of pulmonary embolus can be made based on clinical features, and no further imaging is necessarily required. If no DVT is identified, either ventilation/perfusion (VQ) scanning or CTPA can be used to look for pulmonary emboli. Choice of imaging depends on availability, as well as the balance of radiation to the fetus and to the maternal breast. In both VQ scans and CTPA the radiation exposure to the fetus is very low. A VQ scan has a lower radiation dose to the maternal breast, however if performed postpartum, breastfeeding should be avoided for 12 hours as radioisotope is found in bodily fluids including milk. Modern CT scanners use a very low dose of radiation, so previous concerns about radiation doses to maternal breast tissue leading to an increase in breast cancer risk are likely to no longer be relevant. CTPA imaging can also pick up other pathology within the chest. Both imaging modalities risk being non-diagnostic, CTPA in particular, as the increased cardiac output in pregnancy means the timing of image acquisition (if based on non-pregnant cardiac output calculations) may result in suboptimal opacification of the pulmonary trunk.

3. What treatment would you give her?

First-line treatment in this woman includes high-flow oxygen and intravenous crystalloids. She needs urgent imaging to confirm or refute the suspicion of PE. Other teams who should be involved at an early stage include obstetrics, physicians experienced in managing high-risk PE and intensive care.

It is important to distinguish between high-risk, intermediate-, and low-risk PE, according to the same diagnostic criteria as in non-pregnant individuals. Thrombolysis for high-risk PE should be instituted without delay, and unfractionated heparin rather than LMWH given initially. Surgical embolectomy can be considered if that is a treatment modality readily available. Catheter-directed thrombolysis, if available, has a lower risk of bleeding as the dose of thrombolytic is lower, but this is not yet advocated in any guidelines for management of PE in pregnancy.

In women with low or intermediate-risk PE, LMWH treatment is the treatment, with the use of pregnancy-specific doses and consideration of anti-Xa monitoring. This should be continued for the rest of pregnancy and 6 weeks postnatally, or until at least 3 months of treatment have been given if the VTE occurred late in pregnancy. Where a woman with intermediate-risk PE does not respond to initial LMWH then options include unfractionated heparin, systemic or catheter-directed thrombolysis.

Warfarin is not commonly used for VTE in pregnancy as it is associated with warfarin embryopathy and later in pregnancy with fetal haemorrhage (the fetus has lower vitamin K levels than the mother and a correspondingly higher INR at any given warfarin dose). Direct oral anticoagulants (DOACs) are used frequently outside pregnancy for venous thromboembolism but should be avoided in pregnancy and breastfeeding due to a lack of safety data and suggestions of fetal and infant complications in animal models. Fondaparinux, a synthetic factor Xa inhibitor which does not cross the placenta, is the anticoagulant of choice in women with VTE who cannot tolerate LMWH.

4. What effect does a pulmonary embolism have on the mode of delivery?

The priority in the emergency setting is stabilization of the mother and appropriate resuscitation. Whilst assessment of fetal wellbeing is important, if this is prioritized over resuscitation and treatment of the mother, birth may result in additional maternal morbidity and mortality. A high-risk PE is not an indication for emergency delivery unless there is cardiac arrest. Thrombolysis does not mandate delivery either, as the inevitable operative mode of delivery will further increase bleeding risk. Emergency delivery may be required after thrombolysis if significant haemorrhage occurs, or fetal compromise becomes evident after the maternal condition is stabilized. The timing and mode of birth should be discussed by the multidisciplinary team.

If the woman is haemodynamically stable, or recovers from a high-risk PE without needing delivery, having a pulmonary embolus does not affect the advice about either timing or mode of birth. Neuraxial anaesthesia should be avoided for 24 hours after administration of a therapeutic dose of LMWH, and no further LMWH should be given until at least 4 hours after spinal injection and insertion or removal of an epidural catheter, due to the risk of bleeding within the vertebral canal and compression of the spinal cord. Women should be informed about stopping the LMWH at the time of labour and be advised that if an operative or instrumental birth is required and an insufficient time has passed since the last dose of LMWH, she will require a general anaesthetic. In many centres, induction of labour at term with appropriate LMWH dose timing is offered to women to enable the use of neuraxial techniques and avoid a general anaesthetic.

5. What implication does this diagnosis have for future pregnancies?

The diagnosis of an oestrogen-associated VTE means that she should avoid oestrogen-containing contraceptives in the future. When on therapeutic anticoagulation, effective contraception is recommended to avoid an unplanned pregnancy. She is at increased risk of venous thromboembolism in future pregnancy so should be made aware of this risk, and the need to test for pregnancy regularly if trying to conceive. As soon as the pregnancy test is positive, prophylactic LMWH should be advised, to continue until 6 weeks postnatally.

Further reading

1. RCOG: Reducing the risk of venous thromboembolism during pregnancy and the puerperium (Green-top Guideline No 37a, last updated April 2015). <https://www.rcog.org.uk/globalassets/documents/guidelines/gtg-37a.pdf>
2. RCOG: Thromboembolic Disease in Pregnancy and the Puerperium: Acute Management (Green-top Guideline No 37b, last updated April 2015). <https://www.rcog.org.uk/globalassets/documents/guidelines/gtg-37b.pdf>

Case 36

A 43-year-old woman presented to the Emergency Department at 37 weeks of gestation with central chest and epigastric pain as well as shortness of breath on exertion. She had had similar symptoms intermittently from 20 weeks. She had seen her GP and started antacid therapy. On the day of presentation, the pain and breathlessness had started when she had climbed some stairs but had persisted for an hour when she stopped. She had taken some antacid liquid, but this had not improved her symptoms. At its worst, the pain was 8/10 in severity. She felt nauseated and had vomited once. She felt sweaty and unwell.

This was her third pregnancy. She had been diagnosed with gestational hypertension in her first pregnancy 7 years previously; she had also had gestational hypertension in her second pregnancy and had remained on antihypertensives after that pregnancy. Prior to pregnancy her blood pressure was controlled with low-dose ramipril, which was switched to labetalol after the positive pregnancy test, and at presentation she was taking both labetalol and modified-release nifedipine. She was on no other regular medications. She had a pre-pregnancy BMI of 39 kg/m². She had smoked 10 cigarettes per day from the age of 15 and continued in pregnancy. She did not drink alcohol in pregnancy and did not take any recreational drugs. Her mother had type 2 diabetes mellitus and her father had undergone a coronary artery bypass graft in his 60s following a myocardial infarction.

Initial assessment

General inspection:	GCS 15/15 but unable to complete talk in full sentences due to pain
Heart rate:	96 bpm, regular
Blood pressure:	105/55 mmHg
Respiratory rate:	15 breaths/minute
Temperature:	36.9 °C
Oxygen saturations:	92% on room air
Urinalysis:	No protein

Examination

Cardiovascular:	Normal heart sounds, JVP not raised
Respiratory:	Normal breath sounds throughout
Abdomen:	Soft and non-tender; gravid uterus appropriate size for dates

Bloods

See Table 36.1.

Table 36.1 Bloods

Haemoglobin	111 g/L
WCC	10.3 × 10⁹/L
Platelets	273 × 10⁹/L
Sodium	138 mmol/L
Potassium	4.2 mmol/L
Urea	2.3 mmol/L
Creatinine	55 µmol/L
Bilirubin	9 mmol/L
ALT	11 iU/L
ALP	68 iU/L
Albumin	36 g/L
CRP	6 mg/L
Troponin I	3 pg/ml

Questions

1. What are the possible causes for this presentation?
2. What are the risk factors for ischaemic heart disease in pregnancy?
3. What investigations would you perform?
4. How do you treat acute coronary syndrome in pregnancy?

Answers

1. What are the possible causes for this presentation?

Ischaemic heart disease is responsible for approximately 20% of maternal cardiac deaths, although acute myocardial infarction is relatively uncommon. Atherosclerotic heart disease is the most common cause of heart disease in pregnancy, but more unusual causes of ischaemic heart disease, such as coronary thrombus without atherosclerotic disease, and spontaneous coronary artery dissection, are both more common than outside of pregnancy.

Most cases occur in the third trimester. Clinical presentation can be the same as in non-pregnant individual, including central chest pain, shortness of breath, nausea, and sweating, and clinicians must be careful not to ascribe these symptoms to dyspepsia or reflux.

Women with known coronary artery disease prior to pregnancy are at risk of serious adverse events in pregnancy. It is typically recommended that women wait for at least 1 year after a cardiac event prior to trying to conceive.

Pulmonary embolism can present in a similar way to ischaemic heart disease, with chest pain and shortness of breath, though typically the pain is more pleuritic in nature. As pulmonary emboli can affect cardiac function, ECG changes and a moderate rise in troponin may be observed, which may make it more difficult to distinguish the two aetiologies. More definitive diagnostic tests (such as a CT pulmonary angiogram or ventilation/perfusion scan) are required to diagnose or exclude pulmonary emboli (see Case 35).

Gastro-oesophageal reflux is common in pregnancy. It may be associated with both chest pain, shortness of breath, and a cough, due to acid reflux irritating the vocal cords and pharynx. However, as a diagnosis of acid reflux is often one based only on the history with no confirmatory tests, it should only be made when other significant pathologies have been excluded.

Peptic ulcer disease can occur but is uncommon.

Aortic dissection is more common in pregnancy due to changes in the vascular system. It can present with a variety of symptoms, including with chest, abdominal, and back pain (see Case 1).

Pre-eclampsia can present with retro-sternal or epigastric pain, as well as shortness of breath (at rest or on exertion) or less commonly orthopnoea. These may be the predominant symptoms, though women should also be asked about the more typical symptoms of headache, visual disturbance, and swelling. Pre-eclampsia is more common in women who have pre-existing and/or treated hypertension but can be harder to diagnose. Checking for new-onset proteinuria, as well as renal dysfunction and liver dysfunction, are essential in all unwell pregnant women.

2. What are the risk factors for ischaemic heart disease in pregnancy?

The main risk factors for ischaemic heart disease relating to atherosclerosis are the same in pregnancy as outside of pregnancy, including smoking, family history, pre-existing diabetes, hyperlipidaemia, and hypertension. However, there are additional risk factors for myocardial ischaemia that may occur in pregnancy such as antiphospholipid syndrome and other inflammatory conditions such as lupus, pre-eclampsia and eclampsia, multiparity, sickle cell disease, or cocaine use.

3. What additional investigations would you perform?

Blood tests should be performed including serial troponin measurements (no change to reference range in pregnancy), BNP and coagulation screen. Capillary blood glucose should also be checked and additionally HbA1c if there is any suspicion of underlying pre-existing diabetes.

Imaging including chest radiography is essential in all cases of significant chest pain in pregnancy.

Serial ECGs are also important to look for dynamic changes, remembering that left axis deviation, small Q waves, and T-wave inversion in lead III can all be normal findings in pregnancy.

Echocardiography is advised to look for regional wall motion abnormalities that suggest myocardial ischaemia, evidence of cardiomyopathy, or features of right heart strain.

Additional tests that are readily available and can be considered to help make the diagnosis include:

- A CTPA if a PE is suspected.
- A whole-body CT angiogram if aortic dissection is a potential explanation.
- CT coronary angiography can be used to look for atherosclerotic plaques as well as some coronary artery dissections.
- Exercise testing can be performed in pregnancy, and it is suggested that the target is a submaximal heart rate (80% of predicted) to provoke symptoms if asymptomatic. This is preferable to dobutamine stress tests, which should be avoided if other options are available.
- Cardiac catheterization can be used diagnostically as well as therapeutically in pregnancy. It should be performed by an experienced operator, through a radial approach. The fetal dose of radiation is low.

4. How do you treat acute coronary syndrome in pregnancy?

Management of ischaemic heart disease in pregnancy should ideally be done with a multidisciplinary team including cardiologists, obstetricians, and anaesthetists.

The common medications used to treat ischaemic heart disease are discussed below:

- Low-dose aspirin: safe in pregnancy.
- Clopidogrel: there is little evidence about clopidogrel in pregnancy, but this can be used if aspirin is insufficient or contra-indicated, or if dual antiplatelet therapy is required. Use of neuraxial anaesthesia would usually require treatment cessation for several days.
- Glycoprotein IIb/IIIa inhibitors: not recommended in pregnancy or breast-feeding due to lack of information.
- Beta-blockade: safe in pregnancy, associated with a small reduction in birthweight.
- Recombinant tissue plasminogen activator: safe in pregnancy though with a risk of concomitant bleeding.
- Heparin: both LMWH and unfractionated heparin can be used in pregnancy, and do not cross the placenta. However clinicians must also consider the associated bleeding risk, and the delay required prior to neuraxial anaesthesia in a woman using LMWH.

Therapeutic coronary angiography is safe in pregnancy, though as above should be performed by an experienced operator. Both drug-eluting and bare metal stents have been used in pregnancy for coronary artery disease.

5. How does ischaemic heart disease affect the timing and method of delivery?

The timing and method of delivery should be individualized. Ischaemic heart disease is rarely an indication for delivery, and treatment of an acute myocardial infarction should not be delayed to allow delivery. After an acute myocardial infarction, delivery should ideally be delayed for 2 weeks to ensure optimal management of the mother. Vaginal birth is preferable to caesarean delivery in the absence of other obstetric issues. In women with ongoing angina, an exercise test could be used to aid decision making about mode of birth.

Further reading

1. **V. Regitz-Zagrosek** *et al.* Cardiovascular diseases during pregnancy (management of) Guidelines: The Task Force for the Management of Cardiovascular Diseases during Pregnancy of the European Society of Cardiology (ESC). European Heart Journal. 2018; **39**(34): 3165–241. <https://academic.oup.com/eurheartj/article/39/34/3165/5078465#186437958>

Case 37

A 29-year-old woman in her first pregnancy presented in early labour at 38 weeks of gestation. Her pregnancy had been complicated by nausea and vomiting in the first trimester and heartburn later in pregnancy. She had been well and continued to work as a primary school teacher until the preceding week.

Initial observations were normal and she was admitted to the labour ward. She was progressing well but then started to feel unwell and mentioned this to her midwife. She then started to have a rigor, but her temperature remained normal.

Initial assessment

General inspection: Looks unwell
Heart rate: 140 bpm
Blood pressure: 70/50 mmHg
Respiratory rate: 30 breaths/minute
Temperature: 37.3 °C
Oxygen saturations: 98% on room air
Urinalysis: No protein

Examination

Cardiovascular: Normal heart sounds, no murmurs
Respiratory: Normal breath sounds
Abdomen: Soft and non-tender; no organomegaly; gravid uterus appropriate
                    size for dates.
Neck: No lymphadenopathy
CTG: Fetal tachycardia

Bloods

See Table 37.1.

Table 37.1 Bloods

Haemoglobin	110 g/L
WCC	9.9 × 10⁹/L
Platelets	185 × 10⁹/L
Sodium	134 mmol/L
Potassium	3.6 mmol/L
Urea	1.7 mmol/L
Creatinine	47 µmol/L
Bilirubin	6 µmol/L
ALT	12 iU/L
Albumin	29 g/L
CRP	46 mg/L

Questions

1. What are the possible causes for this acute deterioration?
2. What investigations should be considered?
3. What immediate treatment is required?
4. Are there any specific neonatal considerations?
5. What are the implications of the likely diagnosis on the clinicians caring for her?
6. Where should she be cared for?

Answers

1. What are the possible causes for this acute deterioration?

She has become acutely tachycardic and hypotensive, so several causes of shock need to be considered.

Septic shock is the most likely cause for her deterioration, and the absence of a high temperature does not exclude the diagnosis. The occurrence of a rigor is supportive of sepsis as the likely cause. Sources of sepsis in labour and the postpartum period can include chorioamnionitis, urinary tract infection, lower respiratory tract infection, mastitis, and skin/soft tissue infections. Risk factors for sepsis in pregnancy and the postpartum period include prolonged rupture of membranes, obesity, black or minority ethnic origin, diabetes, anaemia, impaired immunity or immunosuppression, surgical or invasive procedures, vaginal trauma, retained products of conception, intravenous drug use, and Group A streptococcal infection in close contacts.

Common organisms that cause maternal sepsis include Group A beta-haemolytic streptococcus (GAS, *Streptococcus pyogenes*), *Escherichia coli*, *Staphylococcus aureus* and *MRSA*, *Streptococcus pneumonia*, *Clostridium septicus*, and *Morganella morgani*.

GAS is of particular concern in pregnancy as the incidence of this has risen over recent years, accounting for more than 40% of maternal deaths in some series. Pregnant women are 20 times more likely to have an invasive GAS infection than non-pregnant women. GAS infections also often present in clusters within maternity services, which may reflect transmission between patients.

Hypovolaemic shock from bleeding could explain this sudden change, and a normal haemoglobin on the laboratory blood tests does not reassure from this perspective as acute bleeding does not lead to a reduction in haemoglobin until haemodilution has occurred. However, hypovolaemic shock would not explain the rigors.

Cardiogenic shock can also cause this presentation but would not explain the rigor. Other signs of heart failure on clinical examination would be expected.

Obstructive shock (i.e. PE) is another important consideration and can occur at any time in pregnancy.

Anaphylactic shock is also an important potential diagnosis, and her medications should be carefully reviewed with this in mind. Other symptoms and signs (wheeze, tongue/lip swelling, urticarial rash) should also be carefully looked for.

2. What investigations should be considered?

Urgent blood tests should be taken, including blood cultures and coagulation.

Blood gas analysis to give a lactate measurement is also essential in the assessment of an individual with potential septic shock.

Other microbiological samples should be taken, depending on any other symptoms present, including urine for culture, vaginal swab, throat swab (if any symptoms of sore throat), viral PCR for influenza and COVID, or CSF if any meningitic symptoms or signs.

Imaging decisions should be individualized and depend on several factors including progress in labour (may not be appropriate to transfer to a nearby department for imaging), severity of illness, symptoms, and therefore likely source, as well as likelihood of other diagnoses.

Echocardiography may be a useful imaging modality that can be quickly performed at the bedside and may provide important diagnostic information. If an alternative diagnosis is clear, however, such as sepsis, then treatment for this should be started as soon as possible rather than wait for imaging to exclude other diagnoses.

3. What immediate treatment is required?

Recognition of sepsis is key and the topic of several recent media campaigns in the United Kingdom. Maternity early observation warning systems are now commonly used to pick up abnormal physiological parameters which may reflect the onset of sepsis.

Broad-spectrum antibiotics are needed urgently (the target being within an hour of diagnosis), in line with the appropriate local hospital protocol for sepsis in pregnant women. This is usually different to those used in non-pregnant individuals, due to the greater risk of group A streptococcal infection in pregnant women, and therefore the need for the addition of an antibiotic such as clindamycin. Whilst ideally blood cultures should be sent prior to antibiotic administration, the latter should not be delayed whilst waiting for cultures to be taken.

Intravenous fluid resuscitation is also an urgent priority, to address the haemodynamic compromise.

Input from intensive care teams is also likely to be required as there may be little response to fluid resuscitation in severe sepsis, in which case additional treatment such as vasoconstrictors (e.g. noradrenaline) may be required.

Delivery should be considered urgently given the speed of maternal deterioration, and therefore the high risk of fetal compromise as a result.

4. Are there any specific neonatal considerations?

The neonatal team should be involved at birth given the need for close monitoring of the neonate in view of severe maternal infection. Antibiotics for the infant are likely to be required. Further management then depends on the nature of the causative organism if this is identified in the mother.

5. What are the implications of the likely diagnosis on the clinicians caring for her?

GAS infection is the most likely diagnosis in this case. If confirmed on culture, invasive group A streptococcal disease is a notifiable condition in the United Kingdom, as is scarlet fever (the commonest manifestation of group A streptococcal infection in children). It is likely that an assessment of routes of potential acquisition will be required, and consideration of treatment if infected healthcare workers are identified. Broadly, however, the clinicians should be vigilant for any symptoms of streptococcal pharyngitis and remain away from work for 24 hours or more.

6. Where should she be cared for?

It may be that rapid treatment and delivery leads to a rapid stabilization in the maternal condition. However, given the potential for further deterioration and need for close monitoring, she either requires a bed in an obstetric setting where close monitoring can be achieved (including hourly fluid balance, management of arterial line, etc.) or in a high dependency unit setting if this is more appropriate based on local availability of resources.

Further reading

1. RCOG: Bacterial sepsis following pregnancy (Green-top Guideline No 64B, last updated April 2021). <https://www.rcog.org.uk/globalassets/documents/guidelines/gtg_64b.pdf>
2. **A. Leonard** *et al.* Severe Group A streptococcal infections in mothers and their new-borns in London and the south east, 2010–2016: Assessment of risk and audit of public health management. British Journal of Obstetrics and Gynaecology. 2019; **126**(1): 44–53.
3. **J. Steer** *et al.* Guidelines for prevention and control of group A streptococcal infection in acute healthcare and maternity settings in the UK. Journal of Infection. 2012; **64**(1): 1–18.

Case 38

A 37-year-old woman was re-admitted 5 days after birth having developed shortness of breath and wheeze. Her pregnancy had been uncomplicated, and she had required an emergency caesarean section for a failed induction of labour (post-dates). She was discharged 2 days after birth with non-steroidal analgesia and the remainder of a 10-day course of prophylactic LMWH. Daily midwifery review after discharge had not identified any abnormalities except peripheral oedema. She had no other past medical history and no allergies. She was exclusively breastfeeding her infant.

Initial assessment

General inspection:	Unwell, breathless
Heart rate:	90 bpm
Blood pressure:	170/100 mmHg
Respiratory rate:	28 breaths/minute
Temperature:	36.1 °C
Oxygen saturations:	70% on room air (96% on 15 L/min oxygen via non-rebreathe mask)
Urinalysis:	1+ protein

Examination

Cardiovascular:	Normal heart sounds, no murmurs
Respiratory:	Bilateral inspiratory crackles to midzones
Abdomen:	Soft and non-tender. Caesarean section wound healing well, no erythema or exudate
Legs:	Peripheral oedema to knees

Bloods

See Table 38.1.

Table 38.1 Bloods

Haemoglobin	102 g/L
WCC	8.8 × 10^9/L
Platelets	321 × 10^9/L
Sodium	137 mmol/L
Potassium	4.1 mmol/L
Urea	2.9 mmol/L
Creatinine	50 µmol/L
Bilirubin	12 µmol/L
ALT	27 iU/L
Albumin	26 g/L
CRP	65 mg/l

Questions

1. What are the possible causes of this presentation?
2. Do the results of the available blood tests help you diagnostically?
3. What investigations would you arrange?
4. What treatment should be commenced?
5. What do you advise her about future pregnancies?

Answers

1. What are the possible causes of this presentation?

Acute shortness of breath in pregnancy or the postnatal period should always be taken seriously, and a variety of diagnoses need to be considered.

Pulmonary oedema can occur in pregnant and the postpartum period. Her signs are consistent with fluid overload, and there are a variety of cardiogenic and non-cardiogenic causes that need to be considered.

Cardiogenic causes of pulmonary oedema include undiagnosed congenital heart disease and valvular disease, ischaemic heart disease, cardiomyopathy (which may be new and acute e.g. peripartum cardiomyopathy, or long-standing conditions such as an underlying dilated cardiomyopathy).

Pulmonary oedema with a structurally normal heart is more common in pregnancy and causes include iatrogenic fluid overload, recreational drug use, medications (such as tocolytics and non-steroidal agents in particular diclofenac), and pre-eclampsia, which can present for the first time postnatally.

Asthma is often the first diagnosis that is considered when wheeze is reported, however it is well described in pregnancy that pulmonary oedema (and 'cardiac asthma') can be misdiagnosed as asthma, leading to inappropriate treatment and omission of potentially life-saving investigation and intervention. A first presentation of asthma in pregnancy or the postpartum period is very rare and other diagnoses are more likely.

Infection is common, and both viral (e.g. SARS-CoV2 infection) and bacterial infections can occur in pregnant or recently delivered women. A careful assessment for infection is required, with a low threshold for antibiotic treatment.

Pulmonary emboli need to be considered in all women during or after pregnancy who report breathlessness, but this diagnosis does not explain her clinical findings, and it would be unusual for two acute diagnoses to coexist (e.g. pulmonary oedema due to left heart failure and pulmonary embolism). Shortness of breath can be seen in women suspected of having amniotic fluid embolism, however it is unlikely for this to be the only or presenting symptom, particularly at this time postnatally.

Anaemia due to blood loss at birth could cause shortness of breath.

2. Do the results of the available blood tests help you diagnostically?

Her blood tests are reassuring in some respects; she is not profoundly anaemic so this is not a contributor to heart failure or pulmonary oedema, and she has normal kidney function (which can be abnormal in pre-eclampsia). Her CRP is elevated, but this is in keeping with having had a recent caesarean delivery rather than being useful in the diagnosis of infection.

3. What investigations would you arrange?

Blood tests including troponin and BNP may be helpful. Importantly, however, a D-dimer is not useful immediately after birth so this should not be used in the diagnostic assessment. D-dimer use is usually avoided in the first 6 weeks after birth, but many clinicians do not view this as a reliable tool until 12 weeks after birth.

Arterial blood gas is also likely to be useful in this case, both for the values of PaO_2 and $PaCO_2$ to confirm the hypoxia identified on peripheral saturation monitoring, but also for assessing other parameters such as pH which may help with the identification of conditions such as a metabolic acidosis.

Imaging should include a chest radiograph in all women who are short of breath. A chest radiograph requires the use of a very low level of radiation and should be performed as it would be in a non-pregnant individual. Pulmonary oedema is likely if features such as bilateral peri-hilar opacification, upper lobe diversion, pleural effusions, and fluid in the interlobar fissures are present. Pulmonary emboli can cause a variety of changes on the chest radiograph including effusions, wedge-shaped areas of opacification or areas of hypoperfusion. If there is a high suspicion of pulmonary emboli from the history, cross-sectional imaging with CTPA or ventilation-perfusion scan is also required, unless there is a clear alternative diagnosis that can be made on plain chest radiograph (such as infection or pulmonary oedema).

An echocardiogram is an important test that should be performed urgently and was normal in this case.

4. What treatment should be commenced?

Pulmonary oedema is the likely diagnosis in this case, due to either pre-eclampsia or non-steroidal anti-inflammatory use. Diuresis is the important initial treatment and loop diuretics can be used in both pregnancy and breastfeeding. A rapid response to a dose of furosemide would be anticipated which, if associated with an improvement in symptoms, is also helpful if there is doubt about the diagnosis. Any non-steroidal anti-inflammatories should be discontinued. Continuous positive airway pressure can also be used if diuretics are insufficient.

Prophylactic LMWH should be continued when she is an inpatient.

An ACE inhibitor (such as enalapril or captopril given she is breastfeeding) is also an attractive adjunct to treatment, particularly if hypertension is persisting.

5. What do you advise her about future pregnancies?

The risk of recurrence of pre-eclampsia depends on the gestational age of onset of pre-eclampsia in the index pregnancy. Women who develop pre-eclampsia after 37 weeks of gestation have a 13% chance of pre-eclampsia in a subsequent pregnancy, compared to an almost 40% chance in women who have had pre-eclampsia diagnosed before 28 weeks of gestation. The risk of pre-eclampsia can be mitigated by low-dose aspirin (75–150 mg daily), and she should be advised to start this at 12 weeks of gestation in any future pregnancies. She should also be advised to avoid non-steroid anti-inflammatories after any future delivery in case this contributed to her pulmonary oedema.

Further reading

1. **D. Rolnik** *et al.* Aspirin versus placebo in pregnancies at high risk for preterm pre-eclampsia. New England Journal of Medicine. 2017; **377**: 613–22.

2. **D. Mostello** *et al.* Recurrence of preeclampsia: Effects of gestational age at delivery of the first pregnancy, body mass index, paternity and interval between births. American Journal of Obstetrics and Gynaecology. 2007; **199**(1): 55.e1–7.

Case 39

A 23-year-old woman in her first pregnancy presented at 32 weeks of gestation with severe chest pain, shortness of breath, and bilateral lower limb pain. She was known to have sickle cell disease (HbSS), and prior to pregnancy she had had several admissions with vaso-occlusive crises, including two episodes of chest crisis requiring intensive care support. Whilst regular exchange transfusions had been planned in pregnancy, she had not attended for these since 20 weeks of gestation. Her last vaso-occlusive crisis was 5 weeks prior to this presentation, and she had managed this at home with analgesia. She was prescribed regular aspirin, phenoxymethylpenicillin, and folic acid, however she did not take all of these every day. There was a family history of sickle cell disease. She did not smoke.

Initial assessment

General inspection:	Unwell, in pain, breathless
Heart rate:	115 bpm
Blood pressure:	80/60 mmHg
Respiratory rate:	25 breaths/min
Temperature:	37.8 °C
Oxygen saturations:	100% on 15 L/min oxygen via non-rebreathe mask
Urinalysis:	No protein

Examination

Cardiovascular:	Normal heart sounds, no murmurs
Respiratory:	Wheeze throughout
Abdomen:	Soft abdomen, non-tender gravid uterus
Lower limbs:	Soft, tender to palpation, no erythema. No oedema, pedal pulses palpable

Bloods

See Table 39.1.

Table 39.1 Bloods

Haemoglobin	55 g/L
WCC	15.2 × 10⁹/L
Platelets	500 × 10⁹/L
Sodium	138 mmol/L
Potassium	3.7 mmol/L
Urea	2.2 mmol/L
Creatinine	50 μmol/L
Bilirubin	35 μmol/L
ALT	10 iU/L
ALP	100 iU/L
Albumin	28 g/L
CRP	5 mg/L

Questions

1. What is sickle cell disease and how is it inherited?
2. What medications are used to manage sickle cell disease in pregnancy?
3. What are the potential precipitants for this sickle cell crisis?
4. What are the complications of sickle cell disease?
5. What are the maternal and fetal complications of sickle cell disease?
6. How would you treat her when she is having a crisis?

Answers

1. What is sickle cell disease and how is it inherited?

Sickle cell disease is a group of conditions caused by abnormal haemoglobin (HbS) resulting from mutations in the haemoglobin gene. The most severe disease occurs if two copies of this gene are inherited (HbSS), but sickle cell disease of varying severity can occur if HbS is inherited with another abnormal haemoglobin gene including HbC, HbD, or beta-thalassaemia. Carriers of the condition are asymptomatic unless severely hypoxic or dehydrated.

These inherited genes lead to the production of abnormal globin chains. Under certain, deoxygenated conditions, these abnormal chains cause erythrocytes to become distorted and sickle shaped. Distorted erythrocytes haemolyse readily but can also aggregate within microvasculature, causing local injury, haemolysis, and local infarcts. This leads to the diverse manifestations of sickle cell disease include painful vaso-occlusive crises, haemolytic anaemia, acute chest syndrome, stroke, avascular necrosis, pulmonary hypertension, renal dysfunction, retinal disease, leg ulcers, hyposplenism, cholelithiasis, and venous thromboembolism.

Sickle cell disease is one of the most common inherited conditions worldwide, and though most cases are in people of African and Afro-Caribbean origin, international movement means cases are increasingly found in Europe, the United Kingdom, and the United States. All pregnant women in the United Kingdom are screened for haemoglobinopathies with haemoglobin electrophoresis. If they have sickle cell disease, or carrier status is identified, their partner should be offered screening as per National Screening Committee guidelines to determine the risk of having a child affected by sickle cell disease, and prenatal diagnosis offered if indicated, typically by invasive testing (CVS or amniocentesis).

2. What medications are used to manage sickle cell disease in pregnancy?

Women with sickle cell disease may have functional hyposplenism, increasing their risk of infection with encapsulated organisms, so antibiotic prophylaxis should be continued in pregnancy. Medications used to decrease the incidence of painful crises, such as hydroxycarbamide, should be discontinued as they are teratogenic. Iron-chelating agents, such as desferrioxamine, should be avoided in the first trimester but are occasionally used in the second and third trimesters. High-dose folic acid (5 mg daily) should be commenced pre-conception and continued throughout the pregnancy due to the increased demands of chronic haemolysis. Aspirin should be given from 12 weeks of gestation to reduce the risk of pre-eclampsia. Thromboprophylaxis should be considered in all women with sickle cell disease.

3. What are the potential precipitants for this sickle cell crisis?

Vaso-occlusion is commonly precipitated by hypoxia, infection, dehydration, or acidosis, however often no precipitant is identified. Urinary tract infection is common in pregnancy and bacteriuria may be asymptomatic in the early stages.

4. What are the maternal and fetal complications of sickle cell disease?

Maternal complications include:

- *Sickle cell crises* of all types in pregnancy, particularly in the third trimester.
- *Gestational hypertension and pre-eclampsia*, which can have an earlier onset and a more accelerated course.
- *Venous thromboembolism* is 1.5–5 times more common in women with sickle cell disease.
- *Anaemia* can be exacerbated by the dilutional effect of pregnancy, necessitating top-up or exchange transfusions.
- *Increased risk of infection* from encapsulated organisms, particularly puerperal, respiratory, and urinary infections. Hyposplenism can contribute to the development of severe sepsis.
- *Hyperhaemolysis* is a rare complication of transfusion.
- *Development of atypical red cell antibodies* can occur following transfusion and reduce the amount of compatible blood units available to the mother in the future.

Fetal complications include:

- *Stillbirth and miscarriage* (perinatal mortality is increased 6-fold).
- *Intrauterine growth restriction* so regular growth scans are recommended in the third trimester.
- *Preterm birth.*
- *Inheritance of sickle cell disease.*
- *Haemolytic disease of the newborn* can result from transplacental passage of atypical red cell antibodies.

5. How do you manage a woman with sickle cell disease in pregnancy?

Preconception

Contraception and reproduction advice and information should be provided to all women with sickle cell disease from adolescence. Women with SCD should be screened for chronic complications including pulmonary hypertension, retinal disease, hypertension, and renal disease as well as liver dysfunction. Women considering pregnancy should be screened for iron overload as those with iron overload may benefit from iron chelation prior to conception. In addition, vaccination history should be clarified, including meningitis C, *Haemophilus influenzae* Type B, hepatitis B, and influenza, and vaccinations updated if required.

Women with SCD should take folic acid 5 mg daily from pre-conception to 12 weeks of gestation to reduce the risk of neural tube defects. The higher dose is recommended due to the increased rate of haemolysis in SCD.

Hydroxycarbamide should be stopped 3 months prior to conception as it is teratogenic in animal models.

Angiotensin converting enzyme inhibitors and angiotensin receptor blockers used for treatment of *hypertension* should be stopped before conception. If used for treatment of *proteinuria*, and the woman has regular menstrual cycles and tests for pregnancy regularly, it may be appropriate to continue these until a pregnancy test is positive.

During pregnancy

Women with SCD should be managed by a multidisciplinary team, including an obstetrician, specialist midwife, and haematologist interested in SCD. Women should be screened for any associated conditions, such as renal disease or hypertension, if not done in the pre-conception period. Women should be advised of the risks of SCD in pregnancy and should try to avoid typical precipitants of sickle cell crises (e.g. dehydration).

Prophylactic antibiotics should be continued, which are given to protect women with functional hyposplenism from encapsulated organisms. Folic acid should be started if not done pre-conception, while teratogenic medications should be stopped, if not done prior to pregnancy. Iron supplementation should only be given if there is evidence of iron deficiency.

Women should be started on aspirin from 12 weeks of gestation to reduce the risk of pre-eclampsia. Blood pressure and proteinuria should be checked at every antenatal visit.

Thromboprophylaxis should be considered in all women with SCD, and in particular, women who are admitted with a sickle cell crisis must have prophylactic dose LMWH.

Women with SCD should have ultrasound assessment of fetal growth at least every 4 weeks starting at 24 weeks of gestation, and more frequent scans if there are concerns.

Exchange transfusions may be appropriate in pregnancy but advice from a specialist haematologist should be sought. 'Top-up' transfusions may be needed in acute anaemia. All transfusions increase the risk of allo-immunization, and as women with SCD are likely to need multiple transfusions over their lifetime, transfusions should only be performed if necessary.

Where atypical antibodies have been identified, serial measurements of antibody titre are required and referral for fetal medicine assessment for fetal anaemia is needed if above a certain level.

Intrapartum

Sickle cell disease is not a contraindication to vaginal birth, though women with hip replacements due to avascular necrosis may need advice about the most appropriate birthing positions.

Relevant members of the multidisciplinary team must all be informed when labour is established, and continuous fetal monitoring should be performed due to an increased risk of fetal distress. Women should be kept adequately hydrated throughout with oral and/or intravenous fluids.

Postpartum, women must be given adequate venous thromboembolism prophylaxis.

During a sickle cell crisis

Multidisciplinary management is again key. Analgesia must be given rapidly for painful crises based on the woman's self-assessment of the pain. Opioids, if required, should not be denied on account of the pregnancy. Ideally, an individualized management plan for crises should be constructed prior when the woman is well. Pethidine should be avoided due to the associated risk of seizures. Prophylactic LMWH should be given to all women admitted with a crisis. Fluid, oxygen, warmth, laxatives, antibiotics, anti-pruritics, and anti-emetics should also be given as needed. Women should be investigated to find the cause and outcome of a crisis as they would be outside of pregnancy.

In a chest crisis it is important to perform a chest radiograph, arterial blood gas, and, given the high risk of pulmonary embolism in SCD, a low threshold for cross-sectional imaging is required if acute hypoxia is present. Supportive treatment, analgesia, and incentive spirometry is essential, with involvement of critical care teams as needed.

There is also an increased risk of haemorrhage and thrombotic stroke, and this should be investigated in women with SCD who present with neurological symptoms.

Acute anaemia may have several causes, such as acute sequestration, but may also be a consequence of Parvovirus infection which can cause an aplastic crisis and needs treatment with blood transfusion (as well as appropriate infection control measures including isolation).

Nausea and vomiting of pregnancy can precipitate a sickle cell crisis, so women should seek medical assistance urgently.

Further reading

1. **E. Oteng-ntim** *et al.* Management of sickle cell disease in pregnancy. A British Society for Haematology Guideline. British Journal of Haematology. 2021, **194**(6): 980–95 <https://online library.wiley.com/doi/full/10.1111/bjh.17671>

Case 40

A 35-year-old woman presented to the Maternity Assessment Unit at 34 weeks of gestation with a 12-hour history of reduced fetal movements, on a background of three days of right upper quadrant and epigastric pain, and then vomiting. Her pregnancy had been otherwise uncomplicated with a normal blood pressure at booking (110/65 mmHg). She had a family history of pre-eclampsia.

The midwife was unable to auscultate the fetal heart on initial assessment.

Initial assessment

General inspection: Unwell, pale, in pain
Heart rate: 118 bpm
Blood pressure: 150/90 mmHg
Temperature: 36.2 °C
Oxygen saturations: 99%
Urinalysis: 4+ protein, 2+ blood

Examination

Cardiovascular: Normal heart sounds
Respiratory: Normal breath sounds
Abdomen: Gravid uterus, generalised tenderness with peritonism, bowel
                    sounds present; absent fetal heartbeat on auscultation
Fundoscopy: Some arteriolar narrowing

Bloods

See Table 40.1.

Table 40.1 Bloods

Haemoglobin	99 g/L
WCC	15×10^9/L
Platelets	101×10^9/L
Sodium	133 mmol/L
Potassium	4.6 mmol/L
Urea	2.1 mmol/L
Creatinine	110 µmol/L
C reactive protein	46 mg/L
Bilirubin	16 µmol/L
ALT	284 iU/L
ALP	265 iU/L
Albumin	28 g/L

Questions

1. What are the possible causes of her symptoms?
2. What additional investigations would you arrange?
3. What treatment would you start immediately?

Answers

1. What are the possible causes of her symptoms?

Abdominal pain and vomiting are not uncommon in pregnancy. Underlying pathology ranges from the benign (gastro-oesophageal reflux disease, for example) to the concerning (appendicitis, pyelonephritis, etc.) and therefore a careful clinical assessment is crucial.

This woman is clearly unwell with severe abdominal pain, which requires urgent investigation. The intrauterine death reflects the severity of the maternal illness, as underperfusion of the placenta has quickly led to fetal compromise.

Pre-eclampsia should always be considered in pregnant women with abdominal pain, particularly when it occurs in the right upper quadrant. *Placental abruption* is more common in pre-eclampsia and causes abdominal pain.

Liver pathology such as subcapsular haemorrhage (more common in pre-eclampsia and HELLP), hepatic ischaemia, or portal vein thrombosis can cause this presentation, as can capsular stretch or rupture as a result of underlying pathology.

Biliary pathology is common in women of childbearing age; cholecystectomy is the commonest reason for women to require a surgical procedure in the year following childbirth. A range of biliary diseases should be considered:

- Gallstones can cause right upper quadrant pain, but uncomplicated stones would not cause the systemic illness described here.
- Cholecystitis can cause sepsis and acute maternal illness.
- Cholangitis (the cardinal features being jaundice, fever, and right upper quadrant pain) is another cause of an acute illness like this and requires urgent antibiotics and intervention.

Appendicitis can cause abdominal pain in pregnancy, and the location can differ to that classically described in non-pregnant individuals due to the effect of the pregnant uterus on appendix location.

Pyelonephritis is more common in pregnancy and requires urgent investigation and treatment. The pain described in this case does not fit with a renal cause of pain, so this is less likely to explain this presentation.

Artery aneurysm rupture, in particular the splenic artery, is also a rare cause of abdominal pain in pregnancy.

2. What additional investigations would you arrange?

Bloods including coagulation, albumin, glucose, and lactate are essential as these are markers of liver synthetic function. Other tests including LDH, reticulocyte count, and a blood film are crucial to clarify if haemolysis is present. Other screening looking for liver pathology (antibodies for autoimmune liver disease, viral hepatitis serology) should also be considered.

Urine protein:creatinine ratio should be sent given the proteinuria and possibility of HELLP syndrome.

Fetal ultrasound is urgently required given the lack of fetal heart on auscultation and can be done at the bedside. This may also reveal the presence of intra-abdominal free fluid, depending on the competence of the operator.

Abdominal imaging with ultrasound or CT is urgently required when acute abdominal pain is present. Practically, ultrasound is usually the first-line investigation to clarify the presence of gallbladder or hepatic pathology and avoids the use of ionizing radiation. A CT may be required in a woman who is acutely unwell, and in this case concerns about fetal radiation are not justified given the sad demise of the baby prior to imaging being performed. Even if this were not the case, the use of CT can be justified in an emergency.

3. What treatment would you start immediately?

Pain relief should be part of the immediate management; she is likely to require opioids.

Careful fluid balance monitoring is required. Fluid restriction in accordance with local guidelines for hypertensive disease should also be considered.

Antihypertensive agents should be prescribed in accordance with local prescribing policy, but close monitoring of blood pressure is required given the high risk of haemodynamic instability.

Intravenous magnesium sulphate should be prescribed given the risk of eclamptic seizures. Magnesium excretion is reduced with acute kidney injury and so vigilance for signs of toxicity and monitoring of levels is essential.

Although not relevant in this case, administration of *intramuscular steroids* to aid fetal lung maturation may be indicated depending on the assessment of fetal well-being and gestation. Steroids should be prescribed in any case where there is a viable fetus and risk of preterm birth, in keeping with local guidelines. Caution is required with intramuscular injections in women with significant thrombocytopenia or coagulopathy, and occasionally an intravenous equivalent may be more appropriate.

Medications such as prophylactic LMWH should be withheld until more information about the diagnosis is obtained and a plan is made for urgent intervention.

She was given oral labetalol and her blood pressure improved. An abdominal ultrasound confirmed intrauterine fetal death. Additionally there was free fluid in the abdomen, and abnormal appearance of the parenchyma in the superior part of the right lobe of the liver. Subsequent CT showed a large subcapsular haematoma of the liver with disruption of the hepatic capsule and significant free fluid in the abdomen.

Repeat blood tests

See Table 40.2.

Table 40.2 Repeat blood tests

Haemoglobin	88 g/L
WCC	21 × 10⁹/L
Platelets	87 × 10⁹/L
Sodium	135 mmol/L
Potassium	6.7 mmol/L
Urea	6.1 mmol/L
Creatinine	200 µmol/L
Bilirubin	13 µmol/L
ALT	750 iU/L
ALP	265 iU/L
Albumin	28 g/L
CRP	78 mg/L
PT	19 s
APTT	56 s

Arterial blood gas

See Table 40.3.

Table 40.3 Arterial blood gas on room air

pH	7.16
PaO_2	15.7 kPa
$PaCO_2$	2.19 kPa
Bicarbonate	7.8 mmol/L
Lactate	8 mmol/L
Base excess	−22 mmol/L

Questions

4. What is the cause of the bleeding?

5. What management would you recommend?

Answers

4. What is the cause of the bleeding?

Imaging has shown that she has significant hepatic bleeding with resultant capsular rupture leading to intra-abdominal bleeding and subsequent DIC. There are three main causes to consider:

- HELLP syndrome
- Secondary to a structural abnormality, e.g. a haemangioma
- Spontaneous hepatic haemorrhage

Initially it may be difficult to be sure of what the cause of the bleeding is, but ultimately this does not change the management in the acute setting. Direct inspection of the liver at the time of surgery, or subsequent imaging will show if there is a structural abnormality. Careful review of the history and examination features can help clarify the diagnosis of a hypertensive disorder of pregnancy. In the case described here, she had hypertension and proteinuria, but neither of these are essential for the diagnosis of HELLP syndrome. Importantly, hypovolaemia from acute bleeding may mask hypertension which may only become evident after resuscitation.

5. What management would you recommend?

The care of this woman requires a broad multidisciplinary team including obstetricians, intensivists, obstetric anaesthetists, hepatobiliary specialists, and surgeons.

Urgent resuscitation and stabilization are required prior to any imaging or surgical procedures, as there is a greater chance of complications arising if a woman is inadequately resuscitated prior to an intervention. This includes the judicious use of blood products and intravenous fluids, as well as intravenous magnesium sulphate. Meticulous fluid balance assessment and documentation is required, and placement of a urinary catheter is an important part of this.

Invasive monitoring is required, such as an arterial line and/or central venous catheter.

She requires *contemporaneous hysterotomy and exploratory laparotomy* urgently. This requires specialist surgeons as intra-abdominal packing is likely to be required.

Correction of the coagulopathy with appropriate blood products is required alongside resuscitation and surgical intervention.

She needs to be on an intensive care or high dependency unit following the procedure, with close attention paid to consequences of liver injury including coagulation and glycaemic control, as well as fluid balance.

Further reading

1. **Westbrook** *et al.* Pregnancy and liver disease. Journal of Hepatology. 2016; **64**(4): 933–54.
2. **D. Katarey** *et al.* Pregnancy-specific liver disease. Best Practice & Research: Clinical Obstetrics & Gynaecology. 2020; **68**: 12–22.

Case 41

A 28-year-old woman presented to the Emergency Department with a 1-day history of vomiting blood, following 10 days of profuse vomiting. She reported vomiting a large spoonful of bright red blood on 2 occasions over the last day. The first time was at the end of a bout of vomiting and the blood was mixed with vomitus. The second time was before any further vomiting, and she described fresh, bright red blood. She reported vomiting more than 6 times each day, retching many times each day and feeling nauseated for most of the day. She found it increasingly hard to eat and vomited after drinking fluids. She had also experienced some epigastric tenderness for 2 days. She had not opened her bowels for 2 days but prior to that reported normal stool.

Her last menstrual period was 7 weeks prior to this admission, and she had recently had a positive home pregnancy test. She had a termination of pregnancy a year prior to this due to hyperemesis gravidarum. She described a history of gastro-oesophageal reflux and stopped her proton pump inhibitor when she became pregnant. Her only medications at presentation were pregnancy vitamins. She stopped smoking 2 years previously and had not drunk alcohol since her positive pregnancy test. Prior to that she would drink 20 units of alcohol per week.

Initial assessment

General inspection:	Looks unwell with dry lips. Body weight 54 kg (pre-pregnancy 60 kg)
Heart rate:	102 bpm
Blood pressure:	94/54 mmHg
Temperature:	36.5 °C
Oxygen saturations:	98%
Urinalysis:	No protein, 3+ ketones
Urine pregnancy test:	Positive

Examination

Cardiovascular:	Normal heart sounds
Respiratory:	Normal breath sounds
Abdomen:	Soft, diffusely tender in the epigastrium
Rectal examination:	No masses, no blood, normal stool

Bloods

See Table 41.2.

Table 41.2 Bloods

Haemoglobin	121 g/L
WCC	7.5×10^9/L
Platelets	240×10^9/L
Sodium	143 mmol/L
Potassium	3.1 mmol/L
Urea	6 mmol/L
Creatinine	96 µmol/L
Bilirubin	4 µmol/L
ALT	34 iU/L
ALP	62 iU/L
Albumin	29 g/L

Questions

1. What are the potential causes of profound vomiting in pregnancy?
2. What are the potential causes for haematemesis in pregnancy?
3. What complications can arise?
4. What investigations would you arrange for this woman when in the Emergency Department?
5. What treatment would you recommend?
6. What is the PUQE score?

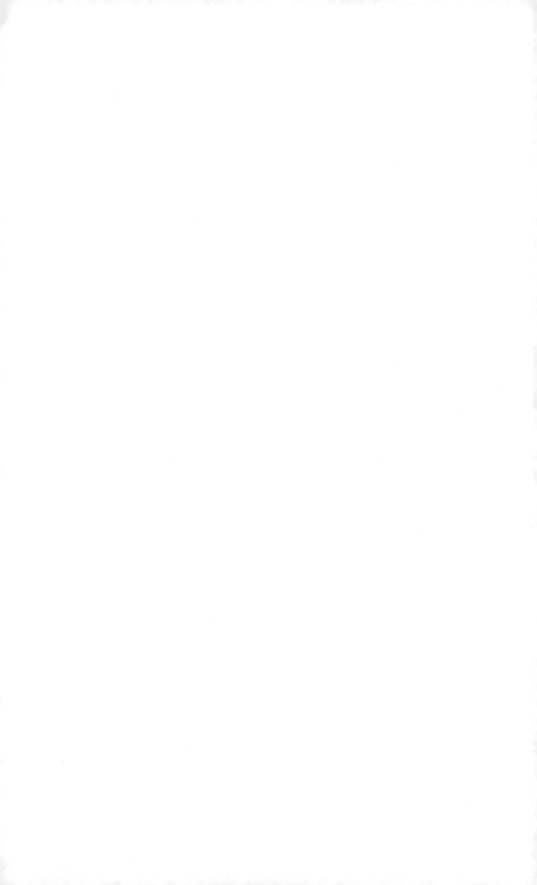

Answers

1. What are the potential causes of profound vomiting in pregnancy?

Hyperemesis gravidarum (HG) is prolonged nausea and vomiting in pregnancy, associated with dehydration, electrolyte imbalance, and more than 5% weight loss from a pre-pregnancy baseline. Nausea and vomiting in pregnancy affect up to 80% of pregnant women, while hyperemesis gravidarum affects up to 4% of pregnant women. HG is more common in women with multiple pregnancy or gestational trophoblastic disease.

Metabolic causes include primary hyperparathyroidism and renal failure.

Infections such as gastrointestinal, urinary tract, and central nervous system infection.

Surgical causes include appendicitis, intestinal obstruction, gastroparesis, cholecystitis, and renal stones.

Neurological causes include migraine, vestibular disorders such as labyrinthitis, and central nervous system conditions such as venous sinus thrombosis.

Gynaecological causes include torsion of ovarian cysts or tumours, or fibroid degeneration. Ectopic pregnancy may present with vomiting.

Drugs and medications can be associated with vomiting, e.g. opioids and cannabis.

2. What are the potential causes for haematemesis in pregnancy?

The most likely cause of haematemesis in this woman is a Mallory–Weiss tear secondary to recurrent vomiting. However, gastritis and oesophagitis are also commonly diagnosed on endoscopy when performed in pregnancy. There are also cases of variceal bleeding and bleeding from gastric tumours that have presented in early pregnancy in association with vomiting.

3. What complications might arise?

Protracted vomiting may result in electrolyte disturbances, teeth damage, oesophagitis, and also rarely oesophageal rupture (Boerhaave syndrome).

Prolonged reduced oral intake can cause complications, e.g. worsening of an underlying medical condition (such as pre-existing diabetes resulting in DKA, or adrenal insufficiency precipitating an adrenal crisis). Other complications such as vitamin deficiency can also develop, so a low threshold for thiamine supplementation particularly should be used.

The structural similarity of HCG and TSH mean it is very common to see biochemical changes suggestive of hyperthyroidism in women with HG. This is known as gestational hyperthyroidism and is not associated with any symptoms of thyroid disease (see Case 2).

4. What investigations would you arrange for this woman from the Emergency Department?

To investigate the haematemesis initial investigations should include a FBC, clotting screen, and urea. An erect chest radiograph can be helpful if perforation is a concern. If the history is not consistent with a Mallory–Weiss tear, an oesophagogastroduodenoscopy should be arranged, which is safe to perform in pregnancy if required. This should be performed by an experienced operator, with the lowest effective dose of sedative. After 20 weeks of gestation, the woman should be positioned in the left lateral position or with a left pelvic tilt to avoid aortic or vena caval compression. When appropriate, the fetal heartbeat should be checked prior to sedation and after the procedure.

To investigate the nausea and vomiting the following tests should be undertaken to look for other causes of symptoms as hyperemesis gravidarum is a diagnosis of exclusion.

Urine	Dipstick, microscopy, and culture
Bloods	FBC, renal function, liver function, amylase, calcium, CRP, thyroid function
Pelvic US	To confirm intrauterine pregnancy, establish viability, and exclude trophoblastic disease or multiple pregnancy
Liver/renal US	If symptoms or blood tests suggest liver or renal pathology

5. What treatment options would you recommend?

Most women with vomiting in pregnancy can be managed on an outpatient basis. Non-pharmacological treatments such as ginger, acupressure, and acupuncture can be tried.

With more severe cases, antiemetics must be used. Antihistamine (H1 receptor antagonists) and phenothiazines are first-line therapies. Metoclopramide can be used as second-line therapy, but women should be informed of the risk of oculogyric crisis. Ondansetron can also be used a second-line therapy. One study showed a small increased risk of cleft palate (3 extra cases per 10,000 births) associated with use in the first trimester, but no increased risk of cardiac anomalies. National guidelines do not view this as an absolute contra-indication to first trimester use, but a discussion of the potential risks and benefits is advised. Combination therapy with drugs of different classes should be used if a first-line treatment fails. Parenteral or rectal antiemetics can also be given.

A combination of doxylamine (an antihistamine) and pyridoxine has recently been licensed for use in pregnancy in the United Kingdom.

Corticosteroids can be used to treat when other therapies have failed, commenced as IV hydrocortisone and, provided there is an improvement in symptoms, switched to oral prednisolone when tolerated and gradually weaned to the lowest effective dose. Diabetes screening is required for women on steroid treatment for over 3 weeks, as well as additional steroid supplementation during intercurrent illness or at delivery.

H2 antihistamines and proton pump inhibitors can be given to reduce the risk of gastro-oesophageal reflux, oesophagitis, and gastritis. The risk of this is increased if steroids are prescribed.

Where available, ambulatory management can be used to review women and treat with intravenous fluids in addition to antiemetics. Inpatient management may be considered if there is:

- Continued nausea and vomiting with an inability to tolerate oral antiemetics.
- Continued nausea and vomiting with persistent weight loss (more than 5% pre-pregnancy body weight) or ketonuria.
- Confirmed or suspected comorbidity e.g. urine infection.

IV rehydration is essential in addition to antiemetics. 0.9% sodium chloride with additional potassium chloride should be first-line therapy, with daily monitoring of electrolytes. Women with HG are at risk of hypo- and hyperkalaemia as well as hyponatraemia.

Oral or intravenous thiamine should also be given to women with prolonged nausea and vomiting who receive ambulatory or inpatient care. Dextrose infusions should be avoided due to the risk of Wernicke's encephalopathy.

Thromboprophylaxis should be given to all women admitted with HG, unless there are specific contraindications.

In protracted and/or severe HG, women should be reviewed by a multidisciplinary team who can provide medical, dietary, and psychological support. Enteral and parenteral nutrition may be appropriate in certain circumstances. In some cases, women may request a termination of pregnancy.

6. What is the PUQE score?

The Pregnancy-Unique Quantification of Emesis (PUQE) Score is a measure of nausea and vomiting in pregnancy. It is a 15-point scale, looking at frequency of nausea, vomiting and retching. It is predominantly used within a research setting but can be used clinically to quantify the severity of nausea and vomiting, though are not predictive of ongoing symptoms. The PUQE score looks at symptoms over 12 hours, while the modified PUQE score looks at symptoms over a typical day.

Further reading

1. RCOG. The management of nausea and vomiting of pregnancy and hyperemesis gravidarum. (Green-top Guideline No 69, last updated June 2016). <https://www.rcog.org.uk/globalassets/documents/guidelines/green-top-guidelines/gtg69-hyperemesis.pdf>
2. A. Lacasse *et al*. Validity of a modified Pregnancy-Unique Quantification of Emesis and Nausea (PUQE) scoring index to assess severity of nausea and vomiting of pregnancy. American Journal of Obstetrics and Gynecology. 2008; **198**(1): 71, e1–7.

Case 42

A 34-year-old woman underwent IVF treatment and became pregnant with DCDA twins. At booking her BP was 117/70 mmHg and her BMI was 28 kg/m². Her pregnancy had been uncomplicated until the diagnosis of gestational diabetes, diagnosed on oral glucose tolerance test at 28 weeks. She was managing her blood glucose levels by dietary changes alone. She presented to the assessment unit at 34 weeks of gestation feeling generally unwell, with symptoms of nausea, alongside new-onset polyuria and polydipsia. She had no past medical history and was not on any regular medication. She was a non-smoker.

Initial assessment

General inspection: Alert, oriented, dehydrated
Heart rate: 90 bpm
Blood pressure: 146/84 mmHg
Respiratory rate: 28 breaths/min
Temperature: 36.6 °C
Oxygen saturations: 99% on room air
Urinalysis: No protein

Examination

Cardiovascular: Normal heart sounds, no murmurs
Respiratory: Normal breath sounds
Abdomen: Mild right upper quadrant tenderness, no peritonism, normal
                    bowel sounds
                    Non-tender gravid uterus
Neurology: Normal

Bloods

See Table 42.1.

Table 42.1 Bloods

Haemoglobin	125 g/L
WCC	21 × 10⁹/L
Platelets	175 × 10⁹/L
Sodium	138 mmol/L
Potassium	5.8 mmol/L
Urea	9 mmol/L
Creatinine	200 µmol/L
Bilirubin	75 µmol/L
ALT	152 iU/L
ALP	254 iU/L
Albumin	17 g/L
CRP	7 mg/L
Amylase	80 U/L
PT	24 s
APTT	45 s
Fibrinogen	2.6 g/L
Blood film	Highly reactive, consistent with acute illness.

Arterial blood gas

See Table 42.2.

Table 42.2 Arterial blood gas

pH	7.27
PaO_2	15.1 kPa
$PaCO_2$	2.4 kPa
HCO_3	13.1 mmol/L
Base excess	−12 mmol/L
Chloride	106 mmol/L
Lactate	4.2 mmol/L
Glucose	3.1 mmol/L

In view of her highly abnormal blood results, and concern about her clinical condition, an emergency caesarean section was performed under general anaesthetic. DCDA twins were delivered in good condition. She was unable to be extubated due to a persistently reduced level of consciousness, so remained intubated and was transferred to ITU for further management.

Questions

1. What potential diagnoses need to be considered here?
2. What is the pathophysiology of this condition?
3. What are the diagnostic criteria?
4. How would you manage this woman?
5. What is her prognosis?

Answers

1. What potential diagnoses need to be considered here?

Acute fatty liver of pregnancy (AFLP) is suggested by her prodromal illness, acute liver injury, and indicators of liver failure (coagulopathy, increased lactate, hypoglycaemia). Whilst the transaminases are not grossly elevated as might be seen in other conditions such as paracetamol-related acute liver injury, this is not uncommon in AFLP and should not deter one from this diagnosis.

AFLP is associated with significant maternal and fetal morbidity and mortality. It is rare, with an approximate incidence of between 1 in 7000 to 1 in 20,000 pregnancies. Potential risk factors for the development of AFLP include fetal long-chain-3-hydroxyacyl-CoA dehydrogenase (L-CHAD) deficiency, multiple pregnancy, low BMI, male fetal sex, previous episode of AFLP, and the development of pre-eclampsia or HELLP syndrome.

The other diagnoses that need to be considered here are *severe pre-eclampsia* and *HELLP syndrome*, the features of which both overlap with that of AFLP.

Other diagnoses to consider include other causes of acute liver failure (viral hepatitis, autoimmune hepatitis, drug-induced hepatitis), as well as obstructive causes of liver failure, including gallstones, and Budd–Chiari syndrome.

2. What is the pathophysiology of this condition?

The pathophysiology of AFLP is not entirely understood. Pathologically, there is microvesicular steatosis of hepatocytes, very different to the macrovesicular steatosis seen in alcohol-related and non-alcohol-related fatty liver disease. In addition, there is little or no inflammation or hepatocellular necrosis.

There has been some association with impaired free fatty acid metabolism, resulting in the accumulation of intermediate metabolites, which subsequently accumulate within maternal hepatocytes and blood with resultant maternal hepatic dysfunction.

Women with AFLP may develop diabetes insipidus. This occurs because there is a reduction in the hepatic metabolism of placental vasopressinase, resulting in increased metabolism of ADH, with a subsequent reduction in circulating ADH. This results in polyuria and polydipsia.

3. What are the diagnostic criteria?

Diagnosis of AFLP is based on a combination of patient symptoms and laboratory findings. The 'Swansea criteria' suggest that the presence of 6 or more of the following is diagnostic for AFLP, importantly in the absence of an alternative diagnosis (Table 42.3).

Liver biopsy, although considered the gold standard for diagnosis, is rarely indicated, or clinically practical, in the presence of coagulopathy. Other imaging modalities include CT and MRI, which may show features of fatty infiltration of the liver, but, equally, may be normal.

Table 42.3 Swansea criteria

Symptoms
Vomiting
Abdominal pain
Polyuria/polydipsia
Encephalopathy
Laboratory
Elevated bilirubin (> 14 µmol/L)
Hypoglycaemia (< 4 mmol/L)
Leucocytosis
Elevated transaminases (> 42 iU/L)
Elevated ammonia (> 47 µmol/L)
Elevated urate (> 340 µmol/L)
Acute kidney injury or creatinine > 150 µmol/L
Coagulopathy or prothrombin time > 14 seconds
Other
Ascites or bright liver on ultrasound scan
Microvesicular steatosis on liver biopsy

4. How would you manage this woman?

The main priorities of management are prompt delivery and maternal support. A multidisciplinary approach should be used, involving obstetricians, anaesthetists, intensivists, neonatologists, and physicians. Patients require monitoring in a high dependency or intensive care environment, due to the potential of acute deterioration and multi-organ involvement. A liver unit should be involved early as, although most patients improve after birth, some may require liver transplantation.

There is no specific treatment (other than delivery), and management focuses on supportive measures. Careful fluid balance monitoring and management is required: excessive and aggressive fluid replacement can lead to pulmonary and cerebral oedema whereas overcautious fluid replacement can worsen acute kidney injury.

Management of hypoglycaemia focuses on careful glucose monitoring and correction of hypoglycaemia with intravenous glucose. *N*-acetylcysteine is increasingly being used in non-paracetamol-related acute liver failure and can be given to women with AFLP. Coagulopathy should be corrected as needed, using intravenous vitamin K and blood products such as fresh frozen plasma.

Patients are at a high risk of developing sepsis so antibiotic prophylaxis should be considered.

5. What is her prognosis?

Most patients recover following birth. Many women decide against future pregnancy because of the severity of the illness they experienced, as recurrence in subsequent pregnancies has been described though it is rare. Recurrence may be more likely in women who are heterozygous for an L-CHAD mutation.

Further reading

1. C. Ch'ng *et al*. Prospective study of liver dysfunction in pregnancy in Southwest Wales. Gut. 2002; 51(6): 876–80.

2. R. Westbrook *et al*. Pregnancy and liver disease. Journal of Hepatology. 2016; **64**(4): 933–45.

Case 43

A 36-year-old woman in her first pregnancy presented to hospital in spontaneous labour at 38 weeks of gestation. She had no past medical history and had taken only simple analgesia prior to labour. Her booking BMI was 38 kg/m². An oxytocin infusion was started for failure to progress, and she had an epidural. Antibiotics were administered as she had previously had a urine sample that showed group B streptococcus. In the moments before birth, she had complained of chest pain and breathlessness and had become increasingly agitated and incoherent. A forceps delivery was performed for fetal bradycardia. Shortly after the birth she became unresponsive with no cardiac output. Cardiac arrest was confirmed, and cardiopulmonary resuscitation was commenced.

Initial assessment

General inspection: Cardiopulmonary resuscitation ongoing
                        One large cannula in left wrist

Vital signs immediately prior to birth
Heart rate: 110 bpm
Blood pressure: 95/45 mmHg
Respiratory rate: 26 breaths/minute
Temperature: 37.8 °C
Oxygen saturations: 93 % on room air

Examination

Cardiovascular: Cool peripheries, pale, no peripheral oedema. Pulses undetectable. Pulseless electrical activity on cardiac monitor.
Respiratory: Bag-valve mask ventilation. Trachea central, bilateral resonant percussion note and breath sounds audible throughout chest with diffuse coarse crepitations.
Abdomen: Soft. Uterus palpable at umbilicus; the placenta had been delivered; copious vaginal bleeding, bimanual compression ongoing.

Venous blood gas

See Table 43.1.

Table 43.1 Venous blood gas

pH	7.25
HCO_3	15 mmol/L
Base excess	−10 mmol/L
Haemoglobin	92 g/L
Potassium	5.1 mmol/L
Sodium	132 mmol/L
Chloride	104 mmol/L
Lactate	4.3 mmol/L

Blood tests

See Table 43.2.

Table 43.2 Blood tests

Haemoglobin	89 g/L
WCC	15.2×10^9/L
Platelets	87×10^9/L
Sodium	134 mmol/L
Potassium	5.0 mmol/L
Urea	2.8 mmol/L
Creatinine	76 μmol/L
Bilirubin	14 μmol/L
ALT	42 iU/L
Albumin	27 g/L
Calcium	2.1 mmol/L
CRP	34 mg/L
INR	1.5
APTT	62 s
Fibrinogen	1.1 g/L

Questions

1. What are the potential causes of this event?
2. What considerations must you make when managing a cardiac arrest in a pregnant woman?
3. How would you manage her?

Answers

1. What are the potential causes of this event?

Life support teaching often refers to the commonest causes of cardiac arrest (hypotension, hypoxia, electrolyte abnormalities, hypothermia, toxins, thrombus, tension pneumothorax, and tamponade) and these should be considered in all settings like that described here. However there are additional pregnancy or delivery-specific causes which are also important.

Amniotic fluid embolism (AFE) is a rare complication of birth that is both difficult to diagnose and treat. Latest estimates from the UK Obstetric Surveillance System are of an incidence of 1.7 per 100,000 pregnancies, a case fatality rate of 0.3 per 100,000 pregnancies and significant morbidity in survivors. Features will usually include acute maternal collapse and/or fetal compromise in labour or immediately after birth, with coagulopathy that is disproportionate to any preceding bleeding. There may be respiratory symptoms, hypotension, confusion, or agitation.

Hypovolaemia secondary to intrapartum bleeding is a common differential diagnosis for AFE as haemorrhage can lead to DIC and collapse. Quantification of bleeding at birth is often found to underestimate actual losses. Some haemorrhage can be concealed within the uterus (placental abruption) or abdomen (broad ligament haematoma, uterine rupture, or bleeding from a distant site such as ruptured aneurysm). It is important to establish whether significant bleeding or blood product replacement preceded the coagulopathy.

Pulmonary embolism is a critical diagnosis to exclude since management is entirely opposite to that of haemorrhage and AFE. PE does not usually generate DIC and bleeding but can cause cardiovascular collapse. Antenatal risk factors for VTE, the circumstances of birth, and whether recent thromboprophylaxis medication has been administered should all be reviewed when evaluating the likelihood of this diagnosis.

Septic shock is another cause of maternal collapse. Maternal sepsis will often manifest insidiously, potentially without the classic hallmarks of a trending tachycardia, fever, and hypotension, due to the patient's physiological reserve and warning signs being mistakenly attributed to normal labour. A raised respiratory rate or fetal tachycardia may be the only preceding markers. Intrapartum observations and potential sources of infection must be carefully reviewed, and all relevant cultures taken. DIC occurs in severe sepsis.

Anaphylaxis must be considered, for which there may be a clear trigger evident from the history (e.g. preceding antibiotics), or other causes such as latex which can be found in bungs used for medication vials. Measurement of mast cell tryptase, whilst not available rapidly enough to be useful in the acute setting, can be helpful in due course in determining whether anaphylaxis was a factor.

Local anaesthetic toxicity can occur as a result of inadvertent intravascular administration of local anaesthetic. If this is thought to have occurred, timely administration of intravenous lipid emulsion can reduce mortality.

Air embolus is most commonly associated with placement of a central venous access device, as air embolus can inadvertently occur following administration of medication or fluid. Presentation is similar to PE, with hypoxia, respiratory compromise, and collapse. Arrhythmias may also occur due to cardiac ischaemia. DIC and bleeding is unusual.

Eclampsia is highly unlikely in this case, but it is important to remember that seizure and collapse can still occur in the context of previously observed normal blood pressure and no protein on urinalysis.

2. What considerations must you make when managing a cardiac arrest in a pregnant woman?

Advanced life support is unchanged in pregnancy, although there are some crucial additional management steps that must be incorporated if the woman is not already delivered.

After 20 weeks of gestation, the gravid uterus will impede circulation by compression of the aorta and inferior vena cava. This can be avoided by either tilting the patient to the left with a wedge or bed tilt, or by lying her flat and manually displacing the uterus to the left. The latter is generally preferable as it facilitates optimum chest compressions.

Preparations must immediately commence to deliver the fetus. A resuscitative hysterotomy (also known as peri-mortem caesarean section) is intended to improve maternal survival by relieving aortocaval compression, alleviating the mechanical hindrance to ventilation by the uterus and reducing the extra oxygen demands required by the pregnancy. It is best practice to have achieved this by the fifth minute of cardiac arrest and should therefore be performed *in situ* rather than waiting for transfer to a sterile theatre environment. If circulation is restored the operation can be completed later with appropriate anaesthesia.

3. How would you manage her?

Initial management in all cases is to follow the Advanced Life Support (ALS) algorithm, taking care to manage the patient's airway, including early intubation with a cuffed endotracheal tube, provide high-flow oxygen, continue cardiopulmonary resuscitation while cardiac output is absent, establish wide-bore intravenous access, and treat shockable rhythms. ALS drugs, doses, and defibrillator energy recommendations are not altered by pregnancy. Although AFE is a diagnosis of exclusion, initial supportive treatment overlaps with many of the differential diagnoses and includes crystalloid fluid and inotropes, uterotonic drugs, and tranexamic acid, alongside the urgent provision of blood products.

Any type of obstetric haemorrhage should be managed with early red cell transfusion. Often there is clinical suspicion of DIC before low fibrinogen or raised PT/APTT is reported, so in this situation early and urgent discussion with the transfusion team should achieve either expedition of sample processing or release of fresh frozen plasma and cryoprecipitate. Platelet pools are also likely to be required.

Recombinant factor VIIa is now only recommended where bleeding persists despite aggressive replacement of coagulation components. Ongoing haemorrhage because of uterine atony may necessitate surgical management steps including intrauterine balloon tamponade, uterine artery ligation or hysterectomy. There are no specific proven treatments for AFE.

Multidisciplinary involvement is essential including the cardiac arrest team, senior anaesthetists, obstetricians, midwives, neonatologists, haematologists, transfusion technicians, and porters. There may be family members present at the birth who will need regular updates and a space to wait in. If circulation is restored, the woman should be managed in an intensive care setting with high-quality communication between teams during transfer, and clear delegation of responsibilities across specialty teams thereafter. Incident reporting, team debrief, and clear documentation of the events must not be forgotten.

In the event of a maternal death, family members and involved staff will require emotional support. The case should be reported to local clinical governance systems, to the coroner/procurator fiscal, to regional and national regulatory bodies, and to MBRRACE-UK.

Further reading

1. **Resuscitation Council**. Adult Advanced Life Support guidelines. (2021). <https://www.resus.org.uk/library/2021-resuscitation-guidelines/adult-advanced-life-support-guidelines>
2. **J. Chu** *et al.* on behalf of the RCOG. Maternal collapse in pregnancy and the puerperium. British Journal of Obstetrics and Gynaecology. 2020; **127**: e14–e52.
3. **S. Paterson-Brown** *et al.* (eds). *Managing Obstetric Emergencies and Trauma* (3rd edn, Cambridge: Cambridge University Press, Cambridge, 2014).

Case 44

A 36-year-old woman attended antenatal clinic at 22 weeks of gestation in her first pregnancy. She had a history of severe rheumatoid arthritis and had required high-dose oral and intra-articular steroids 18 months previously. Prior to pregnancy she was taking methotrexate and a biosimilar TNF-alpha inhibitor. The methotrexate was stopped 2 months prior to conception. Her arthritis had remained quiescent during pregnancy, and she was keen to discuss whether she could stop her TNF-alpha inhibitor.

Questions

1. What effects does pregnancy have on rheumatoid arthritis?
2. What effects does rheumatoid arthritis have on pregnancy?
3. What medications for rheumatoid arthritis are suitable for use in pregnancy?
4. What advice would you give this woman regarding the use of her TNF-alpha inhibitor?
5. What treatment would you offer if she had an acute flare of rheumatoid arthritis in pregnancy?

Answers

1. What effects does pregnancy have on rheumatoid arthritis?

Rheumatoid arthritis improves in pregnancy in approximately 60% of women. Approximately 20% will have a flare of disease during pregnancy requiring further intervention, but more than 30% of all women will have a flare in the postpartum period. Having active disease in early pregnancy, and discontinuation of TNF-alpha inhibitors are both risk factors for disease flare in pregnancy.

2. What effects does rheumatoid arthritis have on pregnancy?

Pregnancy outcomes in women with well-controlled rheumatoid arthritis are similar to those without rheumatoid arthritis. Women with active rheumatoid arthritis, however, are at increased risk of miscarriage, preterm birth, intrauterine growth restriction and small-for-gestational age infants, hypertensive disorders of pregnancy, and caesarean delivery.

3. What medications for rheumatoid arthritis are suitable for use in pregnancy?

Many of the medications used for treatment of rheumatoid arthritis are suitable for use in pregnancy. These include:

- Sulfasalazine (folic acid 5 mg daily needs to be co-prescribed)
- Hydroxychloroquine
- Azathioprine
- TNF-alpha inhibitors (see below)

Some medications however should be avoided due to the risk of teratogenicity. These include:

- Methotrexate
- Leflunomide
- Mycophenolate mofetil
- Cyclophosphamide (in most cases)

4. What advice would you give this woman regarding the use of her TNF-alpha inhibitor?

The TNF-alpha inhibitors are complete or modified IgG1 antibodies that are used to treat immune-mediated inflammatory disorders such as rheumatoid arthritis and inflammatory bowel disease. These are actively transported across the placenta via receptors on syncytiotrophoblasts. This means very little of the inhibitor crosses the placenta in early pregnancy. TNF-alpha inhibitors are therefore safe to use during conception and early pregnancy, and this has been confirmed in large registry studies. Moreover, stopping biological disease-modifying anti-rheumatic drugs ('bDMARDs') is a known risk factor for disease flare in pregnancy, with a potential for worse pregnancy outcomes.

In common with antibodies, transplacental transport of most TNF-alpha inhibitors increases through pregnancy and have been detected in the baby's blood up to 12 months of age. At present, the exception to this is certolizumab, which is a PEGylated fragment of a TNF inhibitor monoclonal antibody and does not cross the placenta. There is no evidence from registry studies that transferred TNF-alpha inhibitors in the baby increases the risk of general infections. However, there was one case report of fatal disseminated Bacille Calmette-Guerin (BCG) infection in a baby aged 3 months whose mother had received high-dose TNF-alpha inhibitor throughout pregnancy. Therefore it is advised that infants born to women on biological therapies should avoid live vaccinations for the first six months of life (with new guidance advocating 12 months in women on infliximab). In the United Kingdom, this affects the schedule of administration of the BCG and rotavirus vaccines in women who were taking biological therapies in the second and third trimesters.

Women with stable rheumatoid arthritis may consider stopping their TNF-alpha inhibitor in the second or third trimesters. Women with unstable disease, or at risk of a significant flare, such as in this case, should be counselled that stopping their medication may exacerbate their symptoms, and given a plan to deal with any flares that do occur. If they continue with the TNF-alpha inhibitor, appropriate communication with primary care is required to ensure the healthcare professionals responsible for the vaccination of the baby are aware of the advice.

Less data are available on the safety in pregnancy of other biological therapies used to treat rheumatoid arthritis, and up-to-date information should be sought for each medication.

5. What treatment would you offer if she had an acute flare of rheumatoid arthritis in pregnancy?

Oral and intra-articular corticosteroids are an effective treatment option for acute flares of rheumatoid arthritis in pregnancy. If needed, intravenous steroids can be given.

Non-steroid anti-inflammatory drugs (NSAIDs) can be safely used in early pregnancy to help with inflammation and pain. Later in pregnancy NSAID use can be associated with premature closure of the ductus arteriosus, which may lead to persistent pulmonary hypertension of the new-born. They may also cause oligohydramnios. Therefore, NSAIDs should be avoided after 28 weeks of gestation.

In women where disease flare or activity is not controlled with their normal medications and corticosteroids, hydroxychloroquine, sulfasalazine, or TNF-alpha inhibitors can all be started in pregnancy.

For pain relief, paracetamol and codeine can be used in all stages of pregnancy, though women must be warned of the constipating effects of codeine.

Further reading

1. **I. Giles** *et al*. Stratifying management of rheumatic disease for pregnancy and breastfeeding. Nature Reviews Rheumatology. 2019; **15**: 391–402.

2. **Mark D Russell** et al, BSR Standards, Audit and Guidelines Working Group, British Society for Rheumatology guideline on prescribing drugs in pregnancy and breastfeeding: immunomodulatory anti-rheumatic drugs and corticosteroids, Rheumatology, 2022. https://doi.org/10.1093/rheumatology/keac551

3. **L. Sammaritano** *et al*. American College of Rheumatology Guideline for the management of reproductive health in rheumatic and musculoskeletal disease. Arthritis and Rheumatology. 2020; 72(4): 529–56.

Case 45

A 32-year-old woman attended the obstetric medicine clinic at 30 weeks of gestation in her first pregnancy. Over the previous 10 weeks, she had been seen three times in the Emergency Department with collapse. She reported that her legs simply gave way and she fell to the ground. She did not lose consciousness, she had no headache, chest pain, palpitations, or any other symptoms. Her arms also felt heavy. Her symptoms improved each time after approximately 30 minutes rest. She had been feeling increasingly fatigued during her pregnancy, particularly in the afternoons, and often had to lie down. In the afternoons, her exercise tolerance had reduced so she could only walk for 10 minutes before feeling completely exhausted and having to rest. She had reduced her oral intake as she felt tired when eating.

Clinical examination on all occasions was normal, including fully cardiovascular and neurological examinations. At the time of one collapse, however, a passer-by reported that she was completely unable to move her limbs for approximately a few minutes. There had been no witnessed seizure activity and no loss of consciousness. Bloods including full blood count, electrolytes, renal function, liver function, thyroid function, and troponin had all been normal, as had an echocardiogram, electrocardiogram, ambulatory ECG monitoring, and an MRI of her head.

She had no other significant medical history and took no regular medication. She did not smoke or drink alcohol.

In clinic, a full autoimmune screen that had been requested following her last Emergency Department attendance was reviewed. She had a high acetyl-choline receptor antibody titre, and a new diagnosis of myasthenia gravis was therefore made.

Questions

1. How does pregnancy affect myasthenia gravis?
2. How does myasthenia gravis affect pregnancy?
3. What treatment can be given for myasthenia gravis in pregnancy?
4. What effects does myasthenia gravis have on the mode and timing of delivery?
5. What effects does myasthenia gravis have on the baby?

Answers

1. How does pregnancy affect myasthenia gravis?

Although myasthenia gravis is a rare autoimmune condition, up to 18% of women experience their first myasthenia symptoms in pregnancy or the first 6 months postpartum. In those with previously diagnosed myasthenia, symptoms worsen in 30–45% of pregnancies. Most exacerbations are mild and myasthenic crises are rare. Exacerbations are most common in the first 6 months postpartum, but often occur when women reduce their regular medications during pregnancy.

2. How dose myasthenia gravis affect pregnancy?

Most women with myasthenia gravis have an uncomplicated pregnancy. There is possibly a slight increase in the risk of preterm rupture of membranes and of miscarriage.

Medications that can exacerbate myasthenia, such as magnesium sulphate, and some antibiotics such as macrolides, should be avoided in women with myasthenia.

3. What treatment can be given for myasthenia gravis in pregnancy?

The acetylcholinesterase inhibitor pyridostigmine can lead to good symptomatic relief and is safe in pregnancy. It can be continued in women with known myasthenia and started in those with a new diagnosis. Intravenous acetylcholinesterase inhibitors should be avoided due to the risk of causing uterine contractions.

Many women require long-term immune suppression. Glucocorticoids (prednisolone), ciclosporin, and azathioprine are appropriate to start or continue in pregnancy, however mycophenolate mofetil and methotrexate should be avoided. Breastfeeding should also be avoided in women taking cyclophosphamide, mycophenolate mofetil, or methotrexate.

Steroid initiation (including steroids for fetal lung maturation) or dose increase should, however, be undertaken with extreme caution, as this can initially worsen myasthenic symptoms.

With worsening symptoms, and particularly if there is a concern about an impending myasthenia crisis, intravenous steroids, and intravenous immunoglobulin or plasma exchange can be used. Respiratory function should be monitored using spirometry to measure vital capacity and maximal inspiratory pressure, and if respiratory function deteriorates, intubation and mechanical ventilation should be considered.

In women who have not had a thymectomy, this should be postponed until after pregnancy as it is unlikely to benefit the woman significantly during pregnancy.

4. What effect does myasthenia gravis have on the mode and timing of delivery?

Women should be advised to deliver in a centre with expertise in managing myasthenia, including neonatal myasthenia, and should be under the care of a multidisciplinary team including an obstetric anaesthetist, neurologist, obstetrician, and neonatologist. The team must also be aware that exacerbations are most common in the postpartum period and that delivery can precipitate a myasthenic crisis.

Myasthenia gravis itself does not affect the timing of birth. Although many case series show a higher rate of caesarean delivery in women with myasthenia, the condition is not itself a contra-indication to vaginal birth, and spontaneous vaginal birth should be encouraged unless there are other obstetric considerations.

In general, neuraxial anaesthesia is preferred to general anaesthesia, and anaesthetists must be aware of which anaesthetics can exacerbate myasthenic symptoms.

Magnesium sulphate is relatively contraindicated in women with myasthenia as it reduces acetylcholine release. Cases where magnesium sulphate may normally be given such as prematurity or pre-eclampsia should be discussed within a multidisciplinary team.

5. What effect does myasthenia gravis have on the baby?

Approximately 10% of babies born to mothers with myasthenia have transient neonatal myasthenia. This presents within 24 hours of birth as weakness, generalized hypotonia, poor sucking, dysphagia, and a weak cry. Rarely there are respiratory complications, but for this reason all infants born to mothers with myasthenia must be reviewed by a neonatologist. Most cases of transient neonatal myasthenia are mild, though some infants do require treatment. It is caused by transplacental transfer of maternal IgG antibodies, and generally resolves within 4 weeks as the antibodies are broken down. There is no correlation between the severity of the maternal myasthenia and the risk of neonatal myasthenia.

A very small number of infants develop arthrogryposis. This is characterized by skeletal abnormalities and joint contractures. Maternal IgG antibodies bind to the fetal type acetylcholine receptors, and reduce fetal movements *in utero*. The importance of awareness of fetal movements should be explained to the mother. Plasma exchange, IVIg, and high-dose steroids can all be used to reduce maternal antibodies if there is a concern about arthrogryposis.

Further reading

1. **D. Sanders** *et al.* International consensus guidance for management of myasthenia gravis. Neurology; 2016; **87**(4): 419–25.
2. N. **Gilhus** *et al.* Myasthenia gravis can have consequences for pregnancy and the developing child. Frontiers in Neurology. 2020; **11**: 554.

Case 46

A 26-year-old woman in her second pregnancy attended the Maternity Assessment Unit at 30 weeks of gestation. She had felt unwell for 1 week, with nausea, malaise, vomiting, transient diarrhoea, mild fever, and non-specific abdominal pain. She also complained of itch on her arms.

She had been well in her pregnancy up to that point. She had no other significant past medical history and was on no regular medication except pregnancy multivitamins. She had been taking paracetamol for the last week to help with her symptoms. She did not drink alcohol and had never smoked. She had not had any unwell contacts. She had spent 1 month in India from 21 weeks of gestation visiting family in both the city and countryside.

Her first pregnancy had been straightforward, and her son had been born at term by an uncomplicated vaginal birth.

Initial assessment

General inspection: GCS 15/15, jaundiced sclerae and skin. No spider naevi. No asterixis.
Heart rate: 102 bpm, regular
Blood pressure: 100/55 mmHg
Respiratory rate: 16 breaths/minute
Oxygen saturations: 98% on room air
Temperature: 37.6 °C
Urinalysis: No protein or glucose

Examination

Cardiovascular: Normal heart sounds, no murmurs
Respiratory: Normal breath sounds
Abdomen: non-tender gravid uterus, appropriate size for dates; 2 cm tender hepatomegaly; no ascites 2 cm mildly tender hepatomegaly, no ascites

Bloods

See Table 46.1.

Table 46.1 Bloods

Haemoglobin	121 g/L
WCC	6.3 × 10⁹/L
Platelets	173 × 10⁹/L
Sodium	138 mmol/L
Potassium	3.6 mmol/L
Urea	2.2 mmol/L
Creatinine	55 µmol/L
Bilirubin	80 µmol/L
ALT	1400 IU/L
ALP	250 IU/L
Albumin	28 g/L
CRP	40 mg/L
Bile acids	45 µmol/L

Questions

1. What are the possible causes for acute liver injury like this in pregnancy?
2. What tests should be performed?
3. How does hepatitis E affect pregnancy?
4. How should a pregnant woman with hepatitis E be managed?

Answers

1. What are the possible causes for acute liver injury like this in pregnancy?

The differential diagnosis of an acute rise in transaminases like this, to over 1000 iU/L is limited to ischaemia, drug-induced liver injury such as paracetamol, and viral hepatitis, in particular hepatitis E. Whilst other causes of a rise in ALT should be considered, such as acute fatty liver of pregnancy, intrahepatic cholestasis of pregnancy and HELLP syndrome need to be considered, it would be unusual for these to cause an ALT of this magnitude (see Cases 22, 40, 42).

Viral hepatitis is a common cause of acute liver failure, particularly in Asian, African, and Far Eastern countries. Possible causes include hepatitis A, B, C, and E, as well as herpes simplex virus (HSV), varicella zoster virus (VZV), Epstein–Barr virus (EBV), adenovirus, and cytomegalovirus (CMV).

Pregnant women are at particular risk of acute failure when exposed to hepatitis E (see more below). Hepatitis E is likely in this case as there is an acute deterioration in liver function, on the background of a non-specific viral illness, and a recent visit to a country where hepatitis E is endemic. The incubation period for hepatitis E infection is approximately 6 weeks. Travel to an endemic area is not essential however, and in the United Kingdom it is possible to contract hepatitis E infection from the ingestion of certain foods such as pork products.

Paracetamol overdose, whether intentional or unintentional, is the most common cause of acute liver failure in the United Kingdom and United States. The maximum dose of paracetamol is the same for pregnant women as for other healthy adults. Unintentional overdose can occur if people take multiple paracetamol-containing products, use medications that affect the CYP2E1 pathway (such as some anticonvulsants) or the CYP450 pathway, have concurrent liver disease and/or chronic alcoholism or if they are significantly malnourished. Paracetamol doses should be calculated in women who are significantly underweight or of very small stature, as the standard adult doses are likely to exceed the maximum recommended dose per weight.

Medications that may be associated with drug-induced liver injury include antibiotics, non-steroidl anti-inflammatories, propylthiouracil, and anticonvulsants. All women presenting with acute liver injury must be asked if they take any herbal or over-the-counter supplements, as well as any routine prescribed medications.

Ischaemic hepatopathy can result from hypoperfusion of the liver and this can occur postpartum if there is significant blood loss, or if blood pressure is reduced too quickly during management of pre-eclampsia.

An acute exacerbation of a previously unknown liver disease such as autoimmune hepatitis or Wilson's disease can cause an acute decline in hepatic function.

2. What tests should be performed?

Blood tests should include routine liver markers (AST, ALT, alkaline phosphatase, gamma-glutamyl transpeptidase (GGT), bilirubin, albumin), and tests of liver synthetic function including lactate, glucose, and coagulation screen. An ammonia level, amylase, lipase, and paracetamol level are also advisable. Other tests to be considered include those for haemolysis, copper levels, and autoimmune screen (antinuclear antibodies, anti-smooth muscle antibodies, anti-liver-kidney-microsome-1 (LKM1) antibodies, anti-liver cytosol antibodies, anti-mitochondrial antibodies, and immunoglobulins).

Viral serology should also be requested urgently, including hepatitis A, B, C, and E, HSV, CMV, EBV, and adenovirus. These can look for evidence of acute, chronic, and past infection. Serum should also be saved for further viral testing if deemed appropriate. For hepatitis E (HEV) infection, anti-HEV IgM appears during early infection, but disappears 4–5 months after the infection. Anti-HEV IgG appears shortly after and can persist for many months or even years. HEV RNA can be detected in both the stool and plasma at the time of acute infection, but it is usually a short-lived viraemia.

Imaging is required, and an ultrasound of the liver and other abdominal organs is the first-line imaging for pregnant women with acute abnormal liver function. This can show hepatomegaly, gross anatomical abnormalities, biliary system structures, and the presence of ascites. CT imaging may be required to look for areas of necrosis as well as at the patency of the hepatic vasculature.

A CT or MRI of the head should be performed in any woman who has evidence of hepatic encephalopathy to rule out other causes of confusion.

A *liver biopsy* is rarely required but should be considered if no other cause for liver dysfunction is found on other non-invasive tests.

3. How may hepatitis E affect pregnancy?

Hepatitis E is endemic in many areas including Asia, India, North Africa, and Mexico. While it can cause liver failure in non-pregnant individuals, pregnant women are at higher risk of severe sequelae, particularly if infected in the second and third trimesters. The underlying reason for this vulnerability is not completely understood but is due to both hormonal and immunological changes that occur in pregnancy.

Maternal complications include:

- *Acute liver failure* affects up to 22% of pregnant women infected with hepatitis E. It results in impaired synthetic function, increasing the risk of bleeding, and can cause hepatic encephalopathy, with subsequent confusion, coma, and death.
- *An increased risk of death* (mortality in pregnancy 15–25% compared to 0.5–3% of non-pregnant individuals).
- *Thrombocytopenia.*
- *Acute kidney injury.*

- *Extrahepatic manifestations* can include glomerulonephritis, pancreatitis, neuro-logical conditions, and mixed cryoglobulinaemia.

  Fetal complications include:
- *Miscarriage, stillbirth, and neonatal death* occur in up to 50% of cases.
- *Prematurity* due to both spontaneous labour and iatrogenic delivery.
- *Infection* as there is up to 50% chance of vertical transmission *in utero*; the virus can also be transmitted through breast milk and nipple lesions, so breastfeeding should be avoided in women who are acutely unwell or have a high viral load.

4. How should a pregnant woman with hepatitis E be managed?

Most cases of hepatitis E are self-limiting and only require supportive management. This includes fluid resuscitation if needed, treatment of hypoglycaemia, and replacement of electrolytes, a proton-pump inhibitor to reduce the risk of gastro-intestinal bleeding, and antibiotics if there is a concern about infection. Blood tests including FBC, electrolytes, ammonia level, coagulation screen, and glucose levels should be checked at least every 6 hours initially.

In non-pregnant individuals, the antiviral ribavirin can be used in some cases, but it is a known teratogen so should be avoided in pregnant women. A hepatitis E vaccine has been developed and approved in China but has not received approval elsewhere in the world and has not been tested in pregnant women.

N-acetylcysteine is safe in pregnancy and may be started while the cause of acute liver failure is being ascertained, and in any case where paracetamol overdose is a possibility.

Hepatic encephalopathy should be treated in a similar way to outside of pregnancy, including regular laxatives and restricted protein intake. Parenteral nutrition may be needed in some situations. Specific techniques to limit cerebral oedema such hyperosmotic medications or hyperventilation can be considered by intensivists.

In rare cases, liver transplant may be indicated.

Further reading

1. **I. Nimgaonkar** *et al*. Hepatitis E virus: advances and challenges. Nature Reviews Gastroenterology & Hepatology. 2018; **15**: 96–110.
2. **C. Wu** *et al*. Hepatitis E virus infection during pregnancy. Virology Journal. 2020; **17**: 73.

Case 47

A 38-year-old woman was found to have low platelets on her booking blood tests in her first pregnancy. This abnormality was confirmed on repeat testing, and she was referred to the specialist clinic for review, where she was seen at 14 weeks of gestation. Her pregnancy had been otherwise uncomplicated. She had no significant past medical history and was taking pregnancy multivitamins. She had never smoked or taken recreational drugs.

Initial assessment

General inspection:	Well; no rashes, bruises, or bleeding
Heart rate:	80 bpm
Blood pressure:	119/67 mmHg
Respiratory rate:	14 breaths/minute
Temperature:	36.6 °C
Oxygen saturations:	99% on room air
Urinalysis:	No abnormalities detected

Examination

Cardiovascular:	Normal heart sounds, no murmurs
Respiratory:	Normal breath sounds
Abdomen:	Soft and non-tender; no organomegaly

Bloods

See Table 47.1.

Table 47.1 Bloods

Haemoglobin	132 g/l
WCC	$7.8 \times 10^9/L$
Platelets	$92 \times 10^9/L$
Haemoglobin electrophoresis	No abnormal variant
PT	12.5 s
APTT	28 s

Questions

1. What are the possible causes of low platelets in pregnancy?
2. What areas in her history should be reviewed to assess her risk of bleeding?
3. What tests would you arrange?
4. What treatment can be offered in pregnancy?
5. What implications do low platelets have for delivery?

Answers

1. What are the possible causes of low platelets in pregnancy?

Thrombocytopenia is defined as a platelet count under 150×10^9/L. It is mild if platelets are over 100×10^9/L, moderate if $50–100 \times 10^9$/l, and severe if under 50×10^9/L. Thrombocytopenia affects approximately 9% of pregnancies. It may be due to increased consumption or destruction of platelets, reduced production of platelets, or dilutional effects. There are pregnancy-specific causes of thrombocytopenia, and other causes unrelated to pregnancy.

Gestational thrombocytopenia accounts for about 75% of cases of thrombocytopenia in pregnancy and is present in 8% of pregnancies. It is typically mild, with platelets in most cases being $130–150 \times 10^9$/L. It usually presents in the second half of pregnancy and resolves spontaneously after birth. A blood count should be performed 6 weeks after childbirth to confirm resolution. There is no bleeding risk to the mother or fetus. It may recur in subsequent pregnancies. There is no specific test for gestational thrombocytopenia, and it is a diagnosis of exclusion.

Hypertensive syndromes (pre-eclampsia/HELLP) account for 15–20% of thrombocytopenia in pregnancy. Thrombocytopenia can be one feature of these systemic disorders of pregnancy, and diagnosis is made by identifying the other features of these conditions.

Folate deficiency can cause thrombocytopenia. Additional features of folate deficiency include macrocytic anaemia, a raised lactate dehydrogenase, and typical features on a blood film including oval macrocytes, hypersegmented granulocytes, and anisopoikilocytosis (see Case 26).

Immune thrombocytopenia (ITP) is the second most common cause of an isolated thrombocytopenia in pregnancy. It affects up to 1% of pregnancies. As with gestational thrombocytopenia, ITP is a diagnosis of exclusion. If not diagnosed prior to pregnancy, it can be hard to distinguish from gestational thrombocytopenia. In general, it is more likely to be ITP if thrombocytopenia is present early in pregnancy, and the diagnosis should be suspected if platelet counts are under 80×10^9/L as this is less common in gestational thrombocytopenia.

Most women are asymptomatic with ITP, but it can cause bleeding from mucous membranes (e.g. petechiae, epistaxis, or gingival bleeding). ITP is caused by antiplatelet antibodies. Maternal IgG antiplatelet antibodies can cross the placenta which can lead to fetal thrombocytopenia. A rare complication of this is fetal intracranial haemorrhage, but the chance of fetal complications does not correlate with maternal platelet count.

Hereditary thrombocytopenias are rare, and there are numerous possible causes with more than 40 responsible genes identified. A family history, including of maternal thrombocytopenia in pregnancy, may suggest hereditary thrombocytopenia. These conditions may be diagnosed prior to pregnancy as they may cause 'platelet-pattern' bleeding, including epistaxis, gingival bleeding, and menorrhagia.

Thrombocytopenia secondary to systemic conditions can also occur, including DIC, the thrombotic microangiopathies including TTP and HUS, bone marrow disorders, and hypersplenism. Diagnosis is made by looking for the other features of these conditions.

Secondary immune thrombocytopenia can be associated with infection (including HIV, hepatitis C, and cytomegalovirus); drug-induced thrombocytopenia (e.g. secondary to heparin, anticonvulsants, and antimicrobials), systemic lupus erythematosus, and antiphospholipid syndrome.

2. What areas in her history should be reviewed to assess her risk of bleeding?

A woman's risk of bleeding can be assessed by reviewing any haemostatic challenges she has previously faced, where she would have been at risk of bleeding. These include:

- Nosebleeds
- Heavy menstrual bleeding
- Bleeding after dental procedures
- Bleeding after any surgery

Any family history of bleeding disorders should also be discussed.

3. What tests would you arrange?

When the diagnosis is not clear from other clinical history and examination, or other laboratory features (e.g. hypertension and proteinuria suggestive of pre-eclampsia), the other following tests are recommended:

- Citrate blood sample for FBC if a blood film shows platelet clumping, which will exclude a low platelet count due to clumping *in vitro*.
- Blood film which will provide information about platelet morphology and other haematological anomalies
- Coagulation screen to exclude other bleeding disorders.

Other more specialized tests to look for hereditary or secondary immune thrombocytopenia may include von Willebrand Factor and Factor VIII levels, thrombogenomics, PFA-100 to look at platelet function, lupus anticoagulant and antiphospholipid antibodies, and ristocetin cofactor activity.

4. What treatment can be offered in pregnancy?

Gestational thrombocytopenia does not require treatment as it does not cause bleeding in the mother or the fetus. The only implication for the mother is whether neuraxial anaesthesia is possible.

Immune thrombocytopenia may need treatment in pregnancy. Criteria for treatment usually used include very severe thrombocytopenia (platelet count under $20 \times 10^9/l$), maternal bleeding or because the woman is near term and requires an increase in platelet count to reduce the likelihood of bleeding at birth or to allow for safe regional anaesthesia. Women with ITP should have their platelet count measured frequently in pregnancy, and weekly towards the time of birth (usually from 32–34 weeks of gestation but local policies vary).

Oral steroids are the first-line treatment and usually result in an increase in platelet number in a few days. Intravenous immunoglobulin (IVIG) can be used if a more rapid response is required or if steroid treatment has failed, with levels increasing in 24–48 hours.

In resistant cases of ITP, IV methylprednisolone, tranexamic acid, rituximab, and azathioprine can also be used. Mothers who are rhesus-D positive and who have an intact spleen are sometimes given anti-D in case this results in an increase in platelet count. Splenectomies have been performed safely in the second trimester to reduce platelet consumption. Platelet transfusions can be used as a temporary measure around the timing of neuraxial anaesthesia and operative or instrumental birth.

Women with ITP should be advised to avoid non-steroidal anti-inflammatories, which is of particular relevance after birth. Women who have previously had a splenectomy should be immunized against pneumococcus, meningococcus, and *Haemophilus influenzae*.

When thrombocytopenia is due to systemic causes or secondary immune thrombocytopenia, the underlying condition should be treated with platelet transfusion cover as required on an individual basis if needed during birth.

5. What implications do low platelets have for delivery?

Thrombocytopenia may affect whether a woman can have a neuraxial block during labour and birth. Low platelets and other bleeding conditions increase the risk of spinal haematoma with subsequent paraplegia. Depending on local policies and expertise, women will need a minimum platelet count of $70–80 \times 10^9/l$ for epidural anaesthesia to be undertaken; some anaesthetists will accept a minimum of $50 \times 10^9/l$ for spinal anaesthesia. Women with low platelets or concerns about bleeding should be assessed by an anaesthetist prior to birth to discuss the alternative options for pain relief during labour, and what would be required in the event of an emergency caesarean delivery. There is also the risk of maternal bleeding with very low platelet counts, but there is no evidence that caesarean delivery is safer or preferable in women with ITP. Platelet transfusions should be considered in women with platelet levels under $50 \times 10^9/l$, depending on local protocols, for both vaginal and operative birth.

In women with ITP (or where the platelet count is low, and the diagnosis of gestational thrombocytopenia is uncertain), various intrapartum interventions are advised against as there is a risk of fetal thrombocytopenia due to transplacental transfer of antiplatelet antibodies. These include placement of a fetal scalp electrode, fetal blood sampling, ventouse birth, and the use of mid-cavity or rotational forceps.

The neonatal team should be informed if the woman has primary or secondary immune-mediated thrombocytopenia, or a hereditary thrombocytopenia, to ensure appropriate investigation and follow-up of the neonate. Umbilical cord blood should be sent for FBC at birth, and if there is thrombocytopenia in the neonate, a sample must be repeated at 3–5 days of life to coincide with the expected nadir in platelet count.

Further reading

1. American College of Obstetrics & Gynaecology Practice Bulletin No. 166: Thrombocytopenia in Pregnancy; Obstetrics & Gynaecology; 2016; **128**(3): e43–e53.

Case 48

A 43-year-old woman with type 2 diabetes mellitus was seen in the antenatal clinic at 9 weeks of gestation in her first pregnancy. This pregnancy was unplanned, and she had never discussed pregnancy or pre-pregnancy counselling with health care professionals. In addition to diabetes, she had a history of hypertension and polycystic ovarian syndrome. Her current medications include metformin, liraglutide, and ramipril. She has no features of diabetic neuropathy or nephropathy and no history of cardiovascular disease.

She attends her first trimester retinal screening which shows proliferative diabetic retinopathy and mild macular oedema.

Initial assessment

General inspection:	GCS 15/15
Heart rate:	96 bpm, regular
Blood pressure:	140/60 mmHg
Respiratory rate:	15 breaths/minute
Temperature:	36.9 °C
Oxygen saturations:	99% on room air
Urinalysis:	2+ glucose

Bloods

See Table 48.1.

Table 48.1 Bloods

Haemoglobin	121 g/L
WCC	6.32 × 10⁹/L
Platelets	273 × 10⁹/L
Sodium	138 mmol/L
Potassium	4.2 mmol/L
Urea	5 mmol/L
Creatinine	55 µmol/L
Bilirubin	5 µmol/L
ALT	45 iU/L
ALP	98 iU/L
Albumin	31 g/L
CRP	6 mg/L
HbA1c	89 mmol/mol

Questions

1. What effects of diabetes on pregnancy should be discussed?
2. What changes would you recommend to her medications?
3. How would you treat her diabetic eye disease in pregnancy?

Answers

1. What effects of diabetes on pregnancy should be discussed with this woman?

There are many potential issues in pregnancy that a woman with diabetes should know about, to be discussed at either pre-pregnancy counselling or the earliest stage possible in pregnancy.

Risks to the baby

Risk of miscarriage is increased in women with diabetes. This is linked to glycaemic control, with increased risk of miscarriage with worsening glycaemic control. If available, women with pre-existing diabetes should be offered an early pregnancy ultrasound scan to confirm viability of the pregnancy.

The incidence of congenital abnormalities is increased; women with pre-existing diabetes have twice the risk of having a baby with congenital abnormalities as a woman without diabetes. Cardiac abnormalities are particularly common, with increasing frequency as HbA1c rises.

Risk of large for gestational age (LGA) baby is increased compared to women without diabetes as increased maternal blood glucose stimulates increased fetal insulin production. This causes increased fat deposition in the fetus, particularly around the abdomen and the shoulders. This can lead to an increased chance of intrapartum complications including failure to progress in labour, shoulder dystocia, and operative delivery (caesarean, forceps, and ventouse).

Risk of preterm delivery is increased due to an increased likelihood of iatrogenic preterm delivery, e.g. related to pre-eclampsia, fetal growth restriction, or LGA growth. Spontaneous preterm birth is more common, and may be secondary to polyhydramnios or preterm, prelabour rupture of membranes.

Risk of stillbirth and neonatal death is increased; women with diabetes are 5 times more likely to have stillbirths. The exact cause for this is unknown but is likely to include placental abnormalities. An increased risk of stillbirth is associated with HbA1c of 48 mmol/mol or above (over 6.5%), being in the highest quintile for deprivation or having type 2 diabetes. In women with pre-existing diabetes and otherwise uncomplicated pregnancy, NICE recommend delivery between 37 weeks and 38 weeks and 6 days of gestation.

Neonatal hypoglycaemia is common when maternal hyperglycaemia is present, due to increased fetal insulin secretion as glucose easily crosses the placenta. The greatest risk is shortly after birth, and the blood glucose of the neonate should be checked regularly prior to feeding during the first few hours of life. Breastfeeding should be encouraged to reduce the chance of hypoglycaemia occurring. Women may also benefit from antenatal colostrum collection to provide additional feeds in the neonatal period. Significant hypoglycaemia may require additional treatment with formula milk or intravenous glucose.

The risk of diabetes in later life is increased, as type 2 diabetes has a strong genetic component. The risk of the infant developing diabetes in later life is 6 times higher if the mother had diabetes. This is likely to be exacerbated by poor glycaemic control during pregnancy.

Risks to the mother

Increased variability in blood glucose control is common, particularly in the first trimester. Women with diabetes should be warned of both hyper- and hypoglycaemic episodes. Nausea, vomiting, and changes in energy levels will contribute to these.

A loss of hypoglycaemic awareness can occur as symptoms of hypoglycaemia may change during pregnancy, which can lead to an increased frequency of hypoglycaemic episodes.

Pre-eclampsia occurs in 15–20% of pregnancies in women with type 1 diabetes, and 10–14% of pregnancies in women with type 2 diabetes, compared to 2–7% of women without pre-existing diabetes. The underlying pathophysiology is not fully understood but may be due to endothelial dysfunction. Women with pre-existing diabetes should therefore take low-dose aspirin from 12 weeks of gestation.

Caesarean delivery is more common in women with pre-existing diabetes, up to 40–70% in some series.

Worsening diabetic retinopathy can occur in pregnancy, with progression occurring in 50–70% of cases. The chance of this occurring is increased in women with a longer duration of diabetes at conception, poor glycaemic control, rapid improvement in glycaemic control, more severe retinopathy at conception, and coexistent hypertension.

Deterioration of diabetic kidney disease may occur, reflected by a worsening in renal function and increase in proteinuria. However uncomplicated pregnancy does not itself cause development of diabetic kidney disease. Renal function and proteinuria may return to baseline levels after pregnancy, but this is less likely in women with chronic kidney disease stages 3–5.

Diabetic ketoacidosis (DKA) is less likely to occur in women with type 2 diabetes. However, it is a serious condition when it occurs in pregnancy and occurs in 0.5–3% of pregnancies in women with type 1 diabetes. It is associated with significant maternal morbidity and mortality as there is dehydration, acidosis, and electrolyte abnormalities which may cause confusion, coma, and cardiac arrest in the mother, as well as affecting uterine perfusion leading to fetal compromise. Pregnant women are more prone to DKA as they are more insulin resistant, have increased counterregulatory hormones, and have a reduced ability to buffer acid due to changes in the respiratory system. Euglycaemic DKA is also more common in pregnancy. The treatment priorities are intravenous insulin, rehydration with 0.9% sodium chloride, and potassium replacement (see Case 14).

2. What changes would you recommend to her medications?

For many women with diabetes, their regular medications need to be changed in pregnancy, and additional medications started to improve pregnancy outcomes.

Women with diabetes are more likely to have a fetus with a neural tube defect, so high-dose folic acid is advised to all women with pre-existing diabetes, ideally 3 months prior to conception and for the first trimester of pregnancy. This woman should therefore be started on high-dose folic acid.

In pregnancy, metformin and insulin are the main treatments for glucose control. Glibenclamide can be used, but this is uncommon in the United Kingdom. Other medications used to lower blood glucose should be stopped, including other sulphonylureas, glucagon-like peptide-1 (GLP1) analogues, dipeptidyl peptidase four (DPP4) inhibitors, and sodium-glucose co-transporter-2 (SGLT2) inhibitors. In this woman, therefore, the liraglutide should be stopped, her metformin dose optimized, and she may require insulin to control her blood glucose as pregnancy progresses.

Angiotensin-converting enzyme (ACE) inhibitors are contra-indicated in the second and third trimesters as they can cause fetotoxicity including renal damage, intrauterine growth restriction, and oligohydramnios. They were previously thought to be teratogenic, but on review of the evidence the association of use in the first trimester and congenital abnormalities is less clear. They should therefore be stopped once a woman knows she is pregnant. If ACE inhibitors are being used to treat hypertension, then labetalol, modified-release nifedipine or methyldopa should be used instead in pregnancy.

Other medications such as statins should also be discontinued.

In view of the increased risk of pre-eclampsia seen in women with pre-existing diabetes, low-dose aspirin (75–150 mg daily) should be started at 12 weeks of gestation.

3. How would you treat her diabetic retinopathy in pregnancy?

Diabetic retinopathy can progress in pregnancy, especially in women who rapidly improve their glycaemic control. Women should have retinal screening in the first trimester of pregnancy unless they had their routine annual retinal screen just prior to conception. If there is no retinopathy, then women should have a further screen at 28 weeks. If there are signs of early diabetic retinopathy at the initial screening, then additional screening should be offered at 16–20 weeks of gestation. The eye drops typically used to dilate the eyes in screening (tropicamide and phenylephrine) are safe in pregnancy. Retinal angiography can be performed in pregnancy if needed.

Pan-retinal photocoagulation is the most common treatment for proliferative diabetic retinopathy and is safe in pregnancy.

Diabetic macular oedema often worsens in pregnancy due to changes in the cardiovascular system and fluid retention. This often improves spontaneously postpartum as these changes resolve. Diabetic macular oedema only therefore occasionally needs treatment during pregnancy. If it is clinically significant and does require treatment, there are several options in pregnancy. Laser therapy can be used if the centre of the macular is not involved. If the centre of the macula is involved, treatment can involve either intra-vitreal steroids or anti-VEGF therapies. VEGF is an essential factor in angiogenesis, so there are theoretical concerns about pregnancy loss and pre-eclampsia, and often therefore intravitreal steroids are preferred, however these also have side effects. There are case series of anti-VEGF use in early pregnancy with no adverse effects reported, so pregnancy is not an absolute contra-indication to its use. A multidisciplinary discussion about alternative options as well as a conversation with the patient about the evidence is therefore important.

Diabetic retinopathy is not a contraindication to vaginal birth.

Further reading

1. W. Amoaku *et al.* Diabetic retinopathy and diabetic macular oedema pathways and management: UK Consensus Working Group Eye. Nature. 2020; **34**: 1–51.
2. NICE. Diabetes in pregnancy: Management from preconception to the postnatal period. 2015. <https://www.nice.org.uk/guidance/ng3>

Case 49

A 41-year-old woman in her first pregnancy was seen in the maternity assessment unit at 34 weeks of gestation. She reported reduced fetal movement for the last 24 hours. She had attended on 2 other occasions for reduced fetal movements in pregnancy, but the CTG had been reassuring each time.

She had been visiting her sister for the last 2 days and her normal antenatal care was in a different hospital. She did not have her maternity notes with her.

She was known to be HIV positive and had been taking highly active anti-retroviral therapy throughout her pregnancy. She reported having an undetectable viral load. She had no other medical conditions and stated her HIV has been well managed since diagnosis. She was also taking pregnancy multivitamins. She had smoked 10 cigarettes per day prior to pregnancy, but gave up when she found she was pregnant.

Initial assessment

General inspection: Alert, oriented, dehydrated
Heart rate: 90 bpm
Blood pressure: 126/84 mmHg
Respiratory rate: 16 breaths/min
Temperature: 36.6 °C
Oxygen saturations: 99% on room air
Urinalysis: No protein

Examination

Cardiovascular: Normal heart sounds, no murmurs
Respiratory: Normal breath sounds
Abdomen: Non-tender gravid uterus, size appropriate for dates
Neurology: Normal

Routine blood tests

See Table 49.1.

Table 49.1 Bloods

Haemoglobin	108 g/L
WCC	7×10^9/L
Platelets	175×10^9/L
Sodium	138 mmol/L
Potassium	3.8 mmol/L
Urea	6 mmol/L
Creatinine	50 μmol/L
Bilirubin	4 μmol/L
ALT	20 iU/L
Albumin	30 g/L
PT	24 s
APTT	45 s
Fibrinogen	2.6 g/L

CTG monitoring is concerning so emergency delivery is considered.

Questions

1. What additional blood tests would you take at this time?
2. What are the guidelines around mode of birth in women with HIV?
3. What advice would you give this woman about breast feeding?
4. What is the risk of transmission of HIV from mother to baby?

Answers

1. What additional blood tests would you take at this time?

Any woman presenting unbooked will be offered blood tests including a FBC. Considering her potential immunocompromised status, it is reasonable to add infection markers, renal, and liver function testing.

Recent blood results from her local unit should also be obtained for comparison.

2. What are the guidelines around mode of birth in women with HIV?

Mode of birth advice for women with HIV centres on the avoidance of vertical transmission to the new-born. If there are no other obstetric considerations, mode of birth depends on gestational age and a woman's viral load.

For women with a viral load measured after 36 weeks of gestation:

- Viral load under 50 HIV RNA copies/ml: planned vaginal birth can be supported, including a vaginal birth after caesarean section (VBAC).
- Viral load of 50–399 HIV RNA copies/ml: pre-labour caesarean section should be considered, but the decision should also take in to account the woman's views, actual viral load and viral load trajectory, length of time on treatment and treatment adherence, and obstetric issues.
- Viral load of 400 or more viral RNA copies/ml: pre-labour caesarean delivery should be recommended.

For a woman who presents in spontaneous labour:

- Viral load under 50 HIV RNA copies/ml: vaginal birth can be supported, with immediate induction or augmentation of labour.
- Viral load of 50–399 HIV RNA copies/ml: immediate caesarean section is recommended, but the decision should also take in to account the woman's views, actual viral load and viral load trajectory, length of time on treatment and treatment adherence, stage of labour, and obstetric issues.
- Viral load of 400 or more HIV RNA copies/ml: immediate caesarean section should be recommended.

3. What advice would you give this woman about breastfeeding?

In the United Kingdom, women with HIV should be advised that formula feeding is the safest way to feed their infant. If the mother decides to breastfeed, however, this can and should be supported. This includes regular review of the mother and infant in clinic including viral load testing in the infant, and maternal combination antiretroviral therapy (cART).

4. What is the risk of transmission of HIV from mother to baby?

In untreated populations, vertical transmission from mother to baby is 25%. In women using combined antiretroviral therapy, and who have an undetectable viral load at birth, transmission rate is 0.3%.

Further reading

1. British HIV Association guidelines for the management of HIV in pregnancy and the postpartum 2018 (2020 third interim update). <https://www.bhiva.org/file/5f1aab1ab9aba/BHIVA-Pregnancy-guidelines-2020-3rd-interim-update.pdf>

Case 50

A 32-year-old woman with multiple sclerosis was referred from a fertility clinic for pre-conception counselling. She had been trying to conceive for 18 months and had regular periods. She had never been pregnant. She was diagnosed with multiple sclerosis 4 years ago, and was initially treated with glatiramer acetate but was switched to natalizumab 2 years ago. She had no relapses in that time.

In addition to monthly natalizumab infusions, she took 4000 units vitamin D daily. She had no other medical conditions.

Questions

1. What effect does multiple sclerosis have on fertility?
2. How does pregnancy affect multiple sclerosis?
3. What supplements are recommended that this woman should start, prior to pregnancy?
4. What advice would you give this woman regarding the use of natalizumab in pregnancy?
5. How can a flare of multiple sclerosis be treated in pregnancy?
6. What advice would you give regarding other disease-modifying therapies for multiple sclerosis in pregnancy?

Answers

1. What effect does multiple sclerosis have on fertility?

Multiple sclerosis (MS) does not affect fertility or the risk of miscarriage. There is thought to be an increased rate of relapses in multiple sclerosis after *in vitro* fertilization (IVF) using gonadotrophin-releasing hormone agonist protocols. The protocol for fertility treatment should therefore be discussed with a fertility specialist.

2. How does pregnancy affect multiple sclerosis?

The risk of MS relapse is reduced in pregnancy, particularly in the third trimester. However, one-quarter of women will have a relapse in the first 3 months postpartum.

Some of the symptoms commonly encountered in normal pregnancy overlap with those of multiple sclerosis, such as fatigue, bladder and bowel symptoms, and carpal tunnel syndrome. Care must be taken to distinguish these symptoms from a relapse.

Women should also be aware that urinary tract infections are common in pregnancy and may exacerbate MS-related symptoms. Women with symptoms of infection should be reviewed promptly with a low threshold for starting antibiotics.

3. What supplements are recommended that this woman should start, prior to pregnancy?

High dose vitamin D is recommended for non-pregnant individuals with MS; the dose does not have to be reduced whilst trying to conceive or in pregnancy.

Women with MS should take folic acid for 3 months prior to conception, and for the first trimester of pregnancy. MS is not an indication for higher dose folic acid supplements.

4. What advice would you give this woman regarding the use of natalizumab in pregnancy?

Women are treated with natalizumab because they have highly active MS, with a high risk of relapse and rebound if natalizumab is stopped. There is minimal transport of natalizumab in the first trimester, and studies show no increased risk of congenital malformation or miscarriage. There is, however, an increased risk of mild, self-limiting haematological disorders in the neonate of women treated with natalizumab. Each woman should therefore be counselled about the risks and benefits of continuing treatment throughout pregnancy. The timing of doses can be adjusted to minimize exposure during the third trimester, but the neonatal team should always be informed. Monitoring for JC virus and progressive multifocal leucoencephalopathy should continue as normal in pregnancy, with lumbar puncture and MRI respectively.

Natalizumab is present in breast milk, but as monoclonal antibodies are digested by the gastrointestinal tract, systemic absorption by the infant is likely to be very small and so natalizumab is not contra-indicated in breastfeeding.

5. How can a flare of multiple sclerosis be treated in pregnancy?

Corticosteroids, either orally or intravenously, are first-line therapy for a flare of multiple sclerosis and are appropriate to use in pregnancy. In severe flares where steroids are ineffective, plasma exchange can be used, with the same indications in pregnancy as in non-pregnant individuals.

6. What advice would you give regarding other disease-modifying therapies for multiple sclerosis in pregnancy?

Glatiramer acetate and interferon-beta preparations are known to be safe in conception and pregnancy. Copaxone®, a form of glatiramer acetate, has a licence for use throughout pregnancy, so may be a preferential preparation for women of reproductive age who are considering pregnancy. Biosimilars of glatiramer acetate exist and are presumed to be as safe as the originator drug, though no studies have proved this yet. If a woman decides to stop glatiramer acetate/interferon-beta preparations in pregnancy, she should be advised that it can take several months for the full efficacy of the drug to return when it is restarted, so she may not be protected from a postpartum relapse. Only small amounts of these glatiramer acetate and interferon-beta pass into breast milk, and no adverse reactions in breastfed infants have been reported, so breastfeeding can be encouraged in women treated with them.

Teriflunomide, fingolimod, and dimethyl fumarate are oral therapies for MS. Teriflunomide is known to be teratogenic and should not be used in pregnancy. It has a long half-life, so women should use effective contraception for the duration of treatment and 2 years afterwards. If a woman is treated with teriflunomide and wishes to become pregnant within 2 years, levels can be reduced faster through an accelerated elimination process. Teriflunomide has been shown to pass to breast milk in animal studies and should be avoided in breastfeeding mothers.

Fingolimod is also teratogenic, and women advised to use effective contraception during treatment and for 2 months afterwards. It is also excreted into breast milk and should be avoided in breastfeeding mothers.

Dimethyl fumarate has not been shown to be teratogenic. However, given the limited data available about its safety in pregnancy, women should be advised to use effective contraception while taking dimethyl fumarate, and potentially switched to an alternative medication if planning to become pregnant. If a woman does become pregnant while using dimethyl fumarate, the decision about whether the benefits of continuing the medication compared to stopping it should be made on an individual basis.

Ocrelizumab and alemtuzumab are both monoclonal antibodies used to treat multiple sclerosis. Neither causes an increased risk of congenital malformations.

However, ocrelizumab can cause B-cell depletion *in utero*, and transient peripheral B-cell depletion and lymphopenia is seen in infants of women on these monoclonal antibodies. Alemtuzumab causes autoimmune disease in 22% of individuals, including autoimmune thyroid disease, immune thrombocytopenic purpura, and Goodpasture's syndrome. For these reasons, women are advised to use effective contraception while being treated with either of these medications.

Women treated with alemtuzumab at any point prior to pregnancy should have thyroid function checked every 3 months during pregnancy, and monthly check of FBC, renal function, and urine to exclude glomerulonephritis. Infants whose mothers were exposed to ocrelizumab during pregnancy should be monitored for B-cell depletion, and live/live-attenuated vaccinations delayed until the infants B-cell count has normalized. Alemtuzumab is found in breast milk, and though the data is lacking, ocrelizumab is likely to be excreted in breast milk as with other humanized IgG antibodies. Due to a lack of safety evidence, these drugs should not be used during breastfeeding, although systemic absorption in the infant is likely to be very low.

Cladribine affects DNA synthesis and is known to be teratogenic. Women are advised to avoid pregnancy for at least 6 months after a course of cladribine. Breastfeeding is also contraindicated while taking cladribine.

Further reading

1. **R. Dobson** *et al.* UK consensus on pregnancy in multiple sclerosis: 'Association of British Neurologists' guidelines. Practical Neurology. 2018; **219**(2): 106–14.
2. **L. Michel** *et al.* Increased risk of multiple sclerosis relapse after in vitro fertilisation. The Journal of Neurology, Neurosurgery and Psychiatry. 2012; **83**(8): 796–802.
3. **R. Dobson** *et al.* Vitamin D supplementation. Practical Neurology. 2018; **18**(1): 35–42.

Case 51

A 30-year-old woman was referred urgently by her GP following a positive pregnancy test. She was originally from Somalia and had previously undergone replacement of her mitral and aortic valves for severe rheumatic heart disease with two mechanical valves. Following the surgery 4 years previously she had been anticoagulated on warfarin, with a stable INR (target 3.0, range 2.5–3.5) on 10 mg warfarin daily. She had been told that she could not conceive on warfarin but had understood that to mean she would be unable to get pregnant, rather than that she should not become pregnant. There had never been concern about valve function. There was no other past medical history, and she was not on any other regular medication. Her BMI was 35 kg/m². She did not smoke or drink alcohol.

Initial assessment

General inspection:	Well
Heart rate:	85 bpm
Blood pressure:	100/65 mmHg
Respiratory rate:	18 breaths/minute
Temperature:	36.1 °C
Oxygen saturations:	99% on room air
Urinalysis:	No protein

Examination

Cardiovascular:	Metallic S1 and S2, quiet systolic murmur, no diastolic murmurs
Respiratory:	Normal breath sounds
Abdomen:	Soft and non-tender; no organomegaly

Bloods

See Table 51.1.

Table 51.1 Bloods

Haemoglobin	112 g/L
WCC	7.8 × 10⁹/L
Platelets	201 × 10⁹/L
Sodium	136 mmol/L
Potassium	3.9 mmol/L
Urea	1.5 mmol/L
Creatinine	47 µmol/L
Bilirubin	6 µmol/L
ALT	12 iU/L
Albumin	28 g/L
INR	3.1

Questions

1. What immediate changes would you make?
2. What risks would you warn her about?
3. How would you counsel her about continuation of pregnancy?
4. What maternal monitoring should be arranged?
5. What fetal monitoring should be arranged?
6. What lessons can be learnt from her history about pre-pregnancy counselling for women with mechanical heart valves?

Answers

1. What immediate changes would you make?

As this is an unplanned and unexpected pregnancy, there are important considerations that she should be advised of, in common with all pregnancies. These include the commencement of folic acid (5 mg daily given her BMI), daily vitamin D supplements, advice about smoking and alcohol if appropriate, and about dietary considerations in pregnancy.

In her case, an early priority is a viability scan, to confirm the pregnancy and approximate gestational age.

As warfarin use in the first trimester can lead to a characteristic embryopathy, changing to LMWH should be discussed. This should be started at an appropriate pregnancy-specific weight-based dose, and anti-Xa monitoring is recommended. This is usually done after the third or subsequent doses. The European Society of Cardiology guidelines suggest that both peak and trough levels are done in women with mechanical valves, with a trough target of 0.6 iµ/ml and peak target of 1.0–1.2 iµ/ml (a slightly lower peak target is advocated if aortic valve replacement alone i.e. 0.8–1.2 iµ/ml). Low-dose aspirin is often started alongside LMWH.

2. What risks would you warn her about?

Pregnancy in women with mechanical heart valves is considered very high risk (WHO risk classification III). Studies show adverse outcomes in 50–70% of pregnancies in women with mechanical valves.

Maternal risks include a risk of valve thrombosis, and mortality associated with this. This is a particular concern when changing anticoagulation, as LMWH is inferior to warfarin in this setting, especially when levels of LMWH are insufficient (as shown by anti-Xa). Counselling about the underlying cardiac condition is also required, as women with metal valves may also have other cardiac pathology, e.g. congenital heart disease, valvular dysfunction, or left ventricular dysfunction.

Fetal risks in the first trimester include miscarriage and warfarin embryopathy, the latter being thought to occur more frequently when the mother requires warfarin doses higher than 5 mg daily. There is therefore a difficult balance to be struck between the risk of embryopathy from first trimester warfarin use, and the risk of thrombosis when an alternative anticoagulant is used. In the second and third trimester, there are risks of fetal bleeding associated with warfarin use, as fetal vitamin K levels are lower than that of the mother, so if the mother has a therapeutic INR, the fetus will have a supratherapeutic INR. Intracranial bleeding is a particular concern as well as fetal loss from retroplacental bleeding. There is also a 0.7–2% chance of fetopathy, with ocular and central nervous system abnormalities.

There are therefore several options that can be used in pregnancy:

1. Warfarin throughout pregnancy

   This is an option for women who are particularly high risk for valve thrombosis or are on low doses of warfarin to maintain a therapeutic INR.

2. LMWH in first trimester, then warfarin from 12 to 36 weeks

   This is a common strategy advocated in women with mechanical heart valves, which recognizes the risk of embryopathy in the first trimester, and the risk of valve thrombosis later in pregnancy if LMWH is used throughout. Warfarin is usually stopped at about 36 weeks, but a little earlier may be appropriate if potential preterm birth is a concern, as it is advised that there is a gap of 2 weeks between stopped warfarin and vaginal birth, due to the risk of fetal bleeding being potentially exacerbated at the time of labour and vaginal delivery.

3. LWMH throughout pregnancy

   Whilst this is an option, it is preferable to reserve this for lower-risk women, e.g. those with modern valves of low thrombogenicity, or aortic valves rather than mitral valves.

Women should be advised about strict adherence to whichever anticoagulant regimen is chosen, and monitoring with anti-Xa or INR is required frequently (every 1–2 weeks) throughout pregnancy.

3. How would you counsel her about continuation of pregnancy?

The woman should be made aware of the high-risk nature of a pregnancy when she has a mechanical valve, so it is appropriate to discuss the risks to her and her baby. Termination of pregnancy is an option that should be discussed with her.

4. What maternal monitoring should be arranged?

The woman requires an echocardiogram to assess valve function as well as other cardiac parameters such as ejection fraction. She also requires regular clinical input about anticoagulation decisions (and later on, birth planning) and anti-Xa monitoring (as above).

5. What fetal monitoring should be arranged?

Whilst the use of warfarin does not affect fetal growth directly, regular fetal surveillance with ultrasound is attractive to identify any bleeding complications, as well as any features which may increase the chance of preterm birth (which may alter the timing of anticoagulation changes). If the underlying maternal cardiac condition was congenital, then a fetal echocardiogram is also advised as there is an increased risk that the infant will also have congenital heart disease.

6. What lessons can be learnt from her history about pre-pregnancy counselling for women with mechanical heart valves?

As in many conditions, pre-pregnancy counselling is crucial. In her case, there was clearly a misunderstanding about the requirement for effective contraception and a lack of explanation about the risks of pregnancy in this setting. Even prior to valve replacement, education in women of childbearing age with valvular lesions is important, to inform them about risks associated with pregnancy, as this may influence the type of valve they choose.

She is changed to LMWH at her first appointment but then returns to warfarin at 12 weeks of gestation. She remains well until 30 weeks when she attends with a small antepartum haemorrhage. A placental abruption is suspected, and urgent caesarean delivery is planned.

Question

7. What do you advise about her anticoagulation?

Answer

7. What do you advise about her anticoagulation?

She is at significant risk of bleeding as she is therapeutically anticoagulated with warfarin. Anti-D immunoglobulin should be administered if her blood group is Rhesus D negative. She requires urgent cross-matching of blood. To reverse the effects of warfarin, intravenous vitamin K and prothrombin complex concentrate should be given. The latter contains factors II, VII, IX, and X and rapidly restores her INR to normal (i.e. within minutes of administration). Vitamin K is given alongside this to maintain the INR as the effect of the prothrombin complex concentrate diminishes over the following hours. The neonatal team should also be informed given the anticoagulated status of the baby.

If there are no haemostatic concerns, a prophylactic dose of LMWH can be given 4–6 hours after birth. Doses are usually increased from day 1 onwards, but recent NICE intrapartum guidelines support the consideration of earlier administration of therapeutic LMWH in women at particularly high risk of valve thrombosis.

Further reading

1. V. Regitz-Zagrosek *et al*. ESC Guidelines for the management of cardiovascular diseases during pregnancy: The Task Force for the Management of Cardiovascular Diseases during Pregnancy of the European Society of Cardiology (ESC). European Heart Journal. 2018; 239(34): 3165–241.
2. NICE. Intrapartum care for women with existing medical conditions or obstetric complications and their babies. NG121. 2019. <https://www.nice.org.uk/guidance/ng121>

Case 52

A 36-year-old woman was seen in a routine antenatal clinic at 28 weeks of gestation in her first pregnancy. She described breathlessness on exertion, extreme fatigue, falling asleep watching TV or reading in a chair, and she had reduced her driving as she is worried about feeling sleepy. She also mentioned that she is concerned her sleep has been poor for a long time (including prior to pregnancy) but had worsened during the second trimester. She described her husband frequently complaining that she snores heavily, and was concerned as he noticed her breathing is somewhat erratic and sometimes there are long pauses. She had no chest pain, cough, or wheeze. She had noticed mild swelling of her ankles bilaterally but no pain or swelling in her calves.

The pregnancy had otherwise been uneventful. Her booking BMI was 45 kg/m² and blood pressure was normal. She had a past medical history of asthma, for which she took an inhaler twice a day and salbutamol when required. She also took a pregnancy multivitamin. She did not smoke.

Initial assessment

General inspection:	Comfortable at rest
Heart rate:	96 bpm
Blood pressure:	126/70 mmHg
Respiratory rate:	15 breaths/min
Temperature:	36.8 °C
Oxygen saturations:	97% on room air
Urinalysis:	No protein

Examination

Cardiovascular:	JVP 4 cm, normal heart sounds, no murmurs
Respiratory:	Normal breath sounds
Abdomen:	Mild epigastric tenderness, non-tender gravid uterus
Legs:	Mild pedal oedema, calves soft and not tender

Arterial blood gas

See Table 52.1.

Table 52.1 Arterial blood gas

pH	7.34
PaCO$_2$	7.1 kPa
PaO$_2$	12.2 kPa
HCO$_3$	30.7 mmol/L

Investigations

CXR   Normal

Questions

1. What are the possible causes of her symptoms?
2. What investigations would you arrange?
3. What effect does the most likely diagnosis have on pregnancy?
4. How should the most likely diagnosis be treated in pregnancy?
5. What other considerations are there for overweight women in pregnancy?

Answers

1. What are the possible causes of her symptoms?

Obstructive sleep apnoea (OSA) is a condition of significant recurrent reduction in airflow during sleep, typically due to upper airway collapse. Some symptoms described here are suggestive of OSA, however breathlessness is less common, so consideration of other potential causes is important.

Obstructive sleep apnoea may be present prior to pregnancy or develop for the first time in pregnancy. The latter is probably due to either weight gain, increased oestrogen causing upper airway oedema, or a combination of influences. It is characterized by pauses in breathing at night, recurrent night-time waking, snoring, and daytime somnolence. OSA in pregnancy is under-recognized and is present in up to 20% of pregnancies in obese women. Risk factors for OSA include older age, obesity, Afro-Caribbean ethnicity, chronic hypertension, and large neck circumference.

Obesity hypoventilation is a cause of type 2 respiratory failure and often overlaps with the features of OSA. Daytime hypercapnia may be present, or simply an abnormally high bicarbonate (reflective of nocturnal type 2 respiratory failure). In contrast to OSA, bilevel non-invasive ventilatory support may be preferable to CPAP.

It is therefore likely that she has an overlap of obesity hypoventilation and obstructive sleep apnoea.

If nocturnal respiratory symptoms are present such as cough and wheeze, other diagnoses such as cardiac failure or asthma need to be considered.

2. What investigations would you arrange?

Arterial blood gas analysis can be helpful in identifying type 2 respiratory failure, which if performed when the patient is awake may be normal apart from a raised bicarbonate. Pregnancy-specific reference ranges should be used when interpreting blood gases, particularly for the partial pressure of CO_2.

Overnight polysomnography is the test of choice to diagnose obstructive sleep apnoea and can be performed in pregnancy in the same way as out of pregnancy and identifies periods of nocturnal hypoxia. The typical screening scores for OSA such as the Epworth Sleepiness scale have significantly reduced sensitivity and specificity in pregnancy, so should not be used.

Echocardiography is indicated if cardiac failure or pulmonary hypertension is suspected. Views can often be suboptimal in pregnancy, and this is worsened in women with severe obesity. If there is significant concern which cannot be adequately assessed on echocardiography alternative imaging such as cardiac MRI is occasionally required.

Peak expiratory flow monitoring can be used in the assessment of asthma.

3. What effect does the most likely diagnosis have on pregnancy?

OSA is associated with significant adverse maternal outcomes, including increased risk of gestational hypertension and pre-eclampsia, gestational diabetes, and caesarean delivery. These risks are independent of maternal age and BMI. There are also adverse fetal outcomes including increased risk of preterm birth and small for gestational age babies.

4. How should the most likely diagnosis be treated in pregnancy?

She is likely to benefit from non-invasive ventilatory support, and this may be bi-level pressure ventilation rather than continuous positive airway pressure given the type 2 respiratory failure pattern on her blood gas.

5. What other considerations are there for overweight women in pregnancy?

Obesity is associated with adverse pregnancy outcomes. For the mother, these include an increased risk of miscarriage, gestational diabetes, pre-eclampsia, venous thromboembolism, dysfunctional or prolonged labour, caesarean section, postpartum haemorrhage, anaesthetic complications, wound infection, postpartum depression, and mortality. Infants of obese women have an increased risk of congenital abnormalities including neural tube defects, macrosomia, preterm birth, stillbirth, and neonatal death. There is also an increased risk of obesity and metabolic disorders in later life.

Obese women will benefit from weight loss prior to conception. During pregnancy all women are advised to eat a healthy diet and maintain exercise, but this is particularly important in women who have a high BMI. Weight loss in obese women in pregnancy can be supported but a severely calorie restricted diet is not advisable as significant weight loss is associated with an increased risk of small for gestational age infants. Weight loss drugs are not recommended in pregnancy.

Women with a BMI of over 30 kg/m^2 are advised to take 5 mg folic acid daily prior to pregnancy and for the first 12 weeks. Obese women are at increased risk of vitamin D deficiency so should be on supplementation in pregnancy. Obesity is a risk factor for pre-eclampsia and BMI over 35 kg/m^2 is one criterion for use of low-dose aspirin in pregnancy. It is also a risk for venous thromboembolism, and obese women may require LMWH in pregnancy depending on BMI, local policy, and other risk factors for VTE. Routine monitoring of anti-Xa levels is supported in RCOG guidelines for VTE treatment for women who are on treatment-dose LMWH and weigh over 90 kg. All women with a BMI over 30 kg/m^2 should be screened for gestational diabetes.

Regular growth scans in the third trimester are often performed in women with obesity to assist in the assessment of fetal growth and presentation as palpation can be less reliable. Anaesthetic review is also required in all women with BMI over 40 kg/m² for airway assessment and consideration of contingencies if neuraxial anaesthesia is required.

Specialist equipment such as bariatric theatre tables, bariatric delivery beds, inflatable transfer mattresses, and hoists may be required for women with a very high BMI.

Further reading

1. RCOG: Care of women with obesity in pregnancy. Green-top Guideline No 72, 2018. <https://www.rcog.org.uk/en/guidelines-research-services/guidelines/gtg72/>

2. Obesity in Pregnancy. American College of Obstetrics & Gynaecology Practice Bulletin, Number 230. 2021; 137(6): e128–144. <https://oce.ovid.com/article/00006250-202106000-00038/HTML>

3. **J. Dominguez** *et al*; Obstructive sleep apnoea in pregnant women: A review of pregnancy outcomes and an approach to management. Anaesthesia & Analgesia. 2018; 127(5): 1167–77.

Case 53

A 45-year-old woman in her first pregnancy presented to the maternity day assessment unit at 22 weeks of gestation with 2 transient episodes of abnormal vision and difficulty speaking normally, associated with a headache. Each episode lasted for about 2 hours, had an acute onset and offset, and had fully resolved by the time she was assessed. She had no past medical history, however had been experiencing unilateral headaches throughout pregnancy. She was not taking any regular medications and had no known drug allergies. Her father had had a stroke aged 60 years. She had never smoked.

Initial assessment

General inspection:	Well in herself
Heart rate:	90 bpm
Blood pressure:	110/80 mmHg
Respiratory rate:	12 breaths/min
Temperature:	36.8 °C
Oxygen saturations:	100% on air
Urinalysis:	No protein

Examination

Cardiovascular:	Normal heart sounds, no murmurs
Respiratory:	Normal breath sounds bilaterally
Abdomen:	Soft abdomen, non-tender gravid uterus
Neurology:	Normal eye movements and cranial nerve examination
	Normal tone, power, coordination, reflexes, and sensation in both upper and lower limbs
Fundoscopy:	Normal

Bloods

See Table 53.1.

Table 53.1 Bloods

Haemoglobin	110 g/L
WCC	9.2 × 10⁹/L
Platelets	210 × 10⁹/L
Na	135 mmol/L
K	3.8 mmol/L
Urea	2.1 mmol/L
Creatinine	40 µmol/L
Bilirubin	7 µmol/L
ALT	10 iU/L
ALP	100 iU/L
Albumin	30 g/L
CRP	3 mg/L

Questions

1. What are the potential causes of her symptoms?
2. What features may help you distinguish between the main potential diagnoses?
3. What important aspects of initial management should be considered?
4. What are the treatment options if her headache was to recur in pregnancy?
5. What causes of ischaemic stroke need to be considered in pregnancy?
6. If an ischaemic event is identified, what other investigations or management options need to be considered?

Answers

1. What are the potential causes of her symptoms?

Migraine is a common cause of transient, stereotypical neurological symptoms and headache and is the most likely diagnosis in this case. The headache is typically unilateral and may be associated with aura (symptoms which precede the migraine, such as visual fortification spectra), photophobia, noise sensitivity (phonophobia), nausea, and vomiting. It is thought to occur secondary to neurovascular inflammation and vasodilation of cerebral blood vessels. There are various types of migraine, including classical migraine (with symptoms described above, and can be associated with neurological symptoms such as aphasia, transient hemianopia, or sensory symptoms), atypical migraine (which may not follow the exact patterns described), and hemiplegic migraine (associated with hemiparesis, and can rarely lead to cerebral infarction). Aura can occur in the absence of a headache. Diagnosis is made on careful history-taking and neurological examination to exclude other causes of headache, such as tension headache, meningitis, cerebral venous sinus thrombosis, amongst others. Imaging is not necessary if the history is typical, however it may be required to exclude other causes.

Migraines can occur for the first time in pregnancy, but the course of migraine in women with a previous history is very variable, and whilst in many the frequency improves in pregnancy, some women experience a significant deterioration in their symptoms.

A *transient ischaemic attack (TIA)* is another cause of transient neurology, resulting from impairment of cerebral blood flow (most commonly secondary to ischaemia as a result of thrombus or other occlusion) to a specific part of the brain, which fully resolves within 24 hours. The symptoms can include speech disturbance, motor and/or sensory impairment, and visual impairment. Headache is much less common. A 'stroke' can present with similar neurological symptoms due to an impaired blood supply to a certain part of the brain, however the abnormalities are present for longer than 24 hours. Strokes occur in 30 in 100,000 pregnancies and are 3 times more common in pregnant than non-pregnant individuals of a similar age. Most pregnancy-related strokes occur in the postpartum period. Ischaemia, haemorrhage, and venous thrombosis may all cause a presentation like this.

A *partial seizure* can cause transient neurological abnormalities, and the exact manifestations depend on the part of the brain involved. This can be followed by signs mimicking a stroke (Todd's paresis).

Multiple sclerosis can cause fluctuating neurological symptoms, however it is uncommon that the symptoms or signs are as short-lived as those described in this case.

Anxiety associated with hyperventilation can produce transient neurology, such as peri-oral tingling, headache, and tremor. It does not tend to have the characteristic symptoms described above.

2. What features may help you distinguish between the main potential diagnoses?

This may be clear from the history if classical features of migraine are present. Sometimes it is difficult, particularly in pregnancy when the nature and frequency of migraine can change, or if transient neurological symptoms occur, such as dysphasia or hemiplegia. Personal history of migraine or seizure can also aid the diagnosis. It should be noted, however, that migraine with aura is associated with an increased lifetime risk of ischaemic stroke.

Traditional risk factors for vascular disease should be considered (hypertension, hypercholesterolaemia, family history, diabetes mellitus, smoking), as these increase the lifetime risk of TIA and ischaemic stroke, but these pathologies can occur in women without any of these risk factors. Additional risk factors for strokes in pregnancy include age over 35 years, pre-eclampsia, and eclampsia as well as underlying medical conditions such as antiphospholipid syndrome, sickle cell disease, thrombotic thrombocytopenic purpura, haemolytic uraemic syndrome, mechanical heart valves, cardiomyopathies and migraine.

3. What important aspects of initial management should be considered?

As her symptoms have resolved, she does not need acute pain relief or empirical medication immediately, however she requires further investigation to clarify the diagnosis.

Imaging such as urgent MRI should be considered given the transient abnormal neurology that she had not experienced on previous occasions, and possibility therefore of an ischaemic event. An urgent MRI will help identify abnormal perfusion on diffusion-weighted imaging which would be consistent with a minor stroke. An MRI is also useful to exclude other structural abnormalities which could cause headache and neurological symptoms. Importantly, a normal MRI does not exclude a transient ischaemic event.

Medication such as aspirin should be considered if a TIA is felt to be a likely diagnosis and the neurological symptoms have fully resolved.

4. What are the treatment options if her headache was to recur in pregnancy?

The management of migraines includes both pharmacological and non-pharmacologic methods, as well as treatment of the acute attack, prevention of further attacks, and management of associated symptoms.

Non-pharmacological interventions include relaxation techniques such as mindfulness, adequate sleep, regular meals, and avoidance of caffeine and other potential precipitants.

Analgesia such as paracetamol and codeine can be used for acute headache relief, but the latter is generally discouraged. Regular use of many analgesics can lead to medication-overuse headache, so it is a difficult balance to achieve. NSAIDs can be used up to 28 weeks of gestation but should be avoided thereafter as there is association with premature closure of the fetal ductus arteriosus.

Antiemetics are an important part of the acute treatment if nausea/vomiting is prominent. Buccal preparations can be helpful. Oral agents such as prochlorperazine or metoclopramide can be used at any point in pregnancy.

Triptans can be used to terminate a migraine in the acute stage. However it is most effective if taken at the start of the migraine, and women are advised to take their triptan as soon as they feel they may be developing a migraine e.g. as soon as they notice a migrainous aura. Whilst tablets are commonly used, effective migraine relief can be achieved rapidly with the use of sumatriptan nasal spray, or buccal rizatriptan.

Preventative treatments should be considered if there are 2 or more disabling headaches per month, use of triptans more than twice per week, migraines with neurological sequelae, or ineffective symptomatic treatment. Options to prevent migraine include propranolol, amitriptyline/nortriptyline, or low-dose aspirin. A greater occipital nerve block can provide effective relief in women with migraine and can be performed in pregnancy. Some treatments should be avoided in pregnancy, such as ergometrine and topiramate.

5. What causes of ischaemic stroke need to be considered in pregnancy?

Ischaemic stroke is rare in women of reproductive age and most commonly occurs as a thromboembolic event in this demographic, as opposed to stenosis or small vessel disease, however these can occur as well. The risk is increased if there are pre-existing risk factors, but the diagnosis should not be dismissed in the absence of these. The risk is higher in the postpartum period.

As in non-pregnant individuals of a young age, it is important to consider secondary causes of ischaemic events, which include:

- Vascular events including vessel dissection, vasculitis, TTP, sickle cell disease, cerebral venous sinus thrombosis
- Prothrombotic states including thrombophilia, antiphospholipid syndrome, and myeloproliferative disorders
- Embolic events, including mitral stenosis, peripartum cardiomyopathy, arrhythmia, endocarditis, paradoxical embolic (e.g. from a patent foramen ovale or atrial septal defect)

6. If an ischaemic event is identified, what other investigations or management options need to be considered?

Given the secondary causes of ischaemic events described above, further investigations including an ECG, echocardiogram, bubble study, carotid Doppler, and autoimmune screen should be considered. Thrombophilia screening may be of value in some cases.

Antiplatelet therapy is an important aspect of treatment if an ischaemic event occurs. The choice of dose and agent depends somewhat on the gestational age and must be individualized.

Aspirin at low dose can be used in pregnancy as normal, but higher doses such as 300 mg daily are usually avoided, especially in the third trimester (concerns similar to NSAIDs i.e. premature closure of the ductus arteriosus). A one-off loading dose of 300 mg is unlikely to cause any problems.

There are less data for clopidogrel in pregnancy, but this is not associated with the same concerns with aspirin in the third trimester. However, clopidogrel has a long half-life and increases the risk of bleeding if given within 7 days of surgery. Therefore the timing and mode of birth must be considered in women on clopidogrel, as it may limit the use of neuraxial analgesia/anaesthesia.

Anticoagulation is usually avoided in the fortnight after an acute ischaemic stroke, even for DVT prophylaxis. It should be reviewed in all women however and considered longer term depending on the likely underlying aetiology, particularly if atrial fibrillation or cardiomyopathy is identified.

Systemic thrombolysis can be used in pregnancy if indicated for acute ischaemic stroke. No randomized studies of thrombolysis in stroke have included pregnant women, so pregnancy and birth are relative contra-indications, and therefore require a multidisciplinary discussion prior to thrombolytic administration. However outcomes are optimal if thrombolysis is administered within 4.5 hours of stroke onset, so discussions must occur promptly.

Thrombectomy can be performed if indicated.

Further reading

1. **A. Khalid** *et al.* A review of stroke in pregnancy: Incidence, investigations and management. The Obstetrician & Gynaecologist. 2020; **22**(10): 21–33.

2. **S. Jarvis** *et al.* Managing migraine in pregnancy. British Medical Journal. 2018; **360**: k80.

3. **K. Grear** *et al.* Stroke and pregnancy: Clinical presentation, evaluation, treatment and epidemiology. Clinical Obstetrics and Gynaecology. 2013; **56** (2): 350–9.

Case 54

A 37-year-old woman presents to the maternity assessment unit at 34 weeks of gestation with a 4-day history of vomiting, dizziness, and fatigue. She had been found to have SARS-CoV2 infection 9 days previously, when she had developed a dry cough, myalgia, and intermittent high fevers. The fevers and cough had stopped 6 days ago but she had continued to feel unwell. She then developed vomiting, fatigue, and dizziness, which had progressively worsened. She did not have any abdominal pain or diarrhoea, had no shortness of breath, cough or coryza, and had no urinary symptoms.

The pregnancy had been unremarkable to that point. She had diagnosed with pulmonary sarcoidosis 3 years prior to pregnancy and had been taking 20 mg of prednisolone daily for the last 18 months. Her only other medications were calcium and vitamin D supplements, omeprazole, and paracetamol when required for fever. She had not been vaccinated against SARS-CoV2. She did not smoke and did not drink alcohol. She had had 1 previous uncomplicated pregnancy which resulted in a spontaneous vaginal birth 8 years previously.

Initial assessment

General inspection:	Unwell, looks dehydrated
Heart rate:	115 bpm
Blood pressure:	102/60 mmHg when lying down, 84/48 mmHg standing
Respiratory rate:	22 breaths/min
Temperature:	37.2 °C
Oxygen saturations:	99% on room air, no desaturation on mobilization
Urinalysis:	No protein

Examination

Cardiovascular:	Normal heart sounds, no murmurs
Respiratory:	Normal breath sounds, no crackles or wheeze
Abdomen:	Soft abdomen, non-tender gravid uterus
Cervix:	Os closed, no sign of rupture of membranes

Bloods

See Table 54.1.

Table 54.1 Bloods

Haemoglobin	110 g/L
WCC	8.7 × 10⁹/L
Platelets	190 × 10⁹/L
Sodium	130 mmol/L
Potassium	5.0 mmol/L
Urea	5.1 mmol/L
Creatinine	60 μmol/L
Bilirubin	8 μmol/L
ALT	20 iU/L
Albumin	28 g/L
CRP	10 mg/L

Nasopharyngeal swab

SARS-CoV2 PCR: detected.

Questions

1. What other aspects of her history are important to consider?
2. What are the possible causes for her symptoms?
3. How would you treat her?

Answers

1. What other aspects of her history are important to consider?

She is on long-term steroids which must not be stopped suddenly as this can lead to adrenal insufficiency. It is therefore important to ask if she has been taking her prednisolone as normal, and whether vomiting has prevented her from doing so. Concerns about immunosuppression from long-term steroids has also led to some individuals stopping their treatment at the time of acute COVID infection, or before, in fear of this contributing to increased severity of illness.

2. What are the possible causes for her symptoms?

An adrenal crisis is the most likely cause for her symptoms. This woman has been on long-term high-dose steroids, and her adrenal axis is likely to be suppressed. An adrenal crisis can produce non-specific symptoms, including nausea, vomiting, exhaustion, myalgia, muscle cramps, abdominal pain, anxiety, and low mood. These symptoms can often be mistaken for normal pregnancy symptoms, particularly in the first trimester. Key examination findings include a significant postural drop (over 20 mmHg difference between lying and standing; important to measure with a manual sphygmomanometer), while biochemically an adrenal crisis may cause hyponatraemia, hyperkalaemia, and hypoglycaemia.

Innate corticosteroid production increases in physiologically normal pregnancies. Therefore pregnant women who are on long-term corticosteroids may need an increase in their dose in pregnancy to avoid an adrenal crisis as they will not be able to increase their own steroid production. Women on long-term steroids should be assessed regularly in pregnancy for signs of steroid deficiency.

SARS-CoV2 infection can cause numerous symptoms including myalgia, nausea, and fatigue and often worsen around day 10 post infection. For further information about SARS-CoV2 infection in pregnancy, see Case 3.

Gastrointestinal infection, either viral or bacterial, may also cause these symptoms.

3. How would you treat her?

Corticosteroid replacement is essential. While she is unwell and vomiting, she should receive 100–200 mg IV or IM immediately, followed by 50 mg hydrocortisone IV/IM every 6 hours. Once she is eating and drinking normally she should restart her 20 mg prednisolone as per 'Sick Day Rules' until she is feeling well again. As she does not have an oxygen requirement, she does not need additional steroid treatment for SARS-CoV2.

Fluid resuscitation with 0.9% sodium chloride is required, to replace fluids lost through vomiting. Careful fluid balance should be instituted.

LMWH for VTE prophylaxis should be given as she is unwell and is an inpatient.

Additional SARS-CoV2 treatment such as monoclonal antibodies or antivirals should be administered as per national guidance and prescribing criteria.

The woman recovered from her acute admission. She had a fetal growth scan at 36 weeks of gestation. This showed an appropriately grown baby, with an estimated fetal weight on the 60th centile. The presentation was breech. On discussion of mode of birth, she declined external cephalic version. She decided to have an elective caesarean section at 39 weeks of gestation, though if she were to labour spontaneously before then she wished to aim for a vaginal breech birth.

Question

4. What advice would you give about steroid coverage around delivery?

Answers

4. What advice would you give about steroid coverage around delivery?

Childbirth is a physiological stressful experience. Extra steroid cover is needed for those women who cannot mount their own adrenal stress response. This includes women who are on physiological replacement doses of steroids (following adrenal failure such as Addison's disease, or following pituitary disease, such as post pituitary surgery), as well as those on long-term oral steroids (equivalent to 5 mg or more prednisolone daily for more than 3 weeks). There is no consensus about how long the risk persists following a course of steroids of 3 weeks or more, so therefore a decision about steroid replacement must be individualized if a woman has had steroids in pregnancy but these were stopped before birth.

These women should continue with their regular oral steroids throughout delivery. Those women having a vaginal birth should receive an extra 50 mg of hydrocortisone IV or IM every 6 hours until 6 hours after the baby is born. Those women who have a planned or emergency caesarean section should have additional IV hydrocortisone at the onset of anaesthesia. If the woman has already had IV or IM hydrocortisone because she was in labour, she would have an additional 50 mg hydrocortisone; if she has not had hydrocortisone in labour, she should have 100 mg hydrocortisone. Women should have a further 50 mg hydrocortisone IV or IM 6 hours post-caesarean section.

Regardless of the mode of birth, if a woman has significant postpartum complications such as major obstetric haemorrhage, IV hydrocortisone should be continued until she is stable and then changed to oral. An increased steroid dose should be given for at least the first 24–48 hours post-delivery, after which she can return to her previous maintenance dose when she is appropriately stable.

Further reading

1. **NICE:** Intrapartum care for women with existing medical conditions or obstetric complications and their babies. (NICE guideline No 121, 2019). <https://www.nice.org.uk/guidance/ng121>
2. **H. Simpson** *et al.* Guidance for the prevention and emergency management of adult patients with adrenal insufficiency. Clinical Medicine. 2020; **20**(4): 371–8.1.

Case 55

A 28-year-old woman with no past medical history was pregnant for the first time. She booked with her midwife at 9 weeks of gestation. Her blood pressure and BMI were normal, and she was scheduled for midwifery-led care. She has been taking pregnancy vitamins for more than 3 months prior to conception. Her booking bloods, however, were significantly abnormal and she was referred for further review in clinic.

Initial assessment

General inspection:	Well but pale. Normal BMI
Heart rate:	94 bpm
Blood pressure:	100/60 mmHg
Temperature:	36.4 °C
Oxygen saturations:	99%
Urinalysis:	No protein or blood

Examination

Neck, axillae:	No lymphadenopathy
Cardiovascular:	Normal heart sounds
Respiratory:	Normal breath sounds
Abdomen:	Soft, non-tender, no organomegaly

Bloods

See Table 55.1.

Table 55.1 Bloods

Haemoglobin	69 g/L
MCV	70 fL
WCC	10 × 10⁹/L
Platelets	350 × 10⁹/L
Sodium	134 mmol/L
Potassium	3.7 mmol/L
Urea	1.6 mmol/L
Creatinine	55 μmol/L
Bilirubin	10 μmol/L
ALT	13 iU/L
ALP	76 iU/L
Albumin	30 g/L
Haemoglobinopathy screen	No abnormality detected

Questions

1. What further aspects of her history would you like to ask about?
2. What additional tests would you suggest?
3. Would your approach be different if she was in the third trimester rather than first?
4. What are the potential consequences for the pregnancy?

Answers

1. What further aspects of her history would you like to ask about?

This woman is profoundly anaemic, with microcytic red blood cells as shown by the low MCV. The main causes of this to consider in pregnancy include iron deficiency, haemoglobinopathies or anaemia of chronic disease. Other causes such as sideroblastic anaemia (inherited or acquired e.g. as a result of lead toxicity) and iron metabolism disorders are extremely rare.

Given these potential causes, a careful history is required, to enquire about bleeding history prior to pregnancy, in particularly menorrhagia, or any other history of blood loss. In the absence of bleeding, malabsorptive causes of iron deficiency such as coeliac disease need to be considered, so questions about family and personal history of autoimmune disease are crucial, as well as establishing whether any other symptoms or consequences of malabsorption are present such as weight loss. The results of the haemoglobinopathy screen sent at booking is also a key part of the assessment, to establish whether a haemoglobinopathy such as thalassaemia is a possible cause of these abnormalities.

It is also important to enquire early as to whether administration of blood products is acceptable to the patient. If this was not, e.g. she declined blood products for religious reasons, then this may require a different management strategy.

2. What additional tests would you suggest?

As a minimum, she requires blood tests for iron studies, folate, and B12. Additional tests performed at the outset depend on the additional history, e.g. if a bleeding history is elicited, coagulation should be assessed. A low threshold for investigations for coeliac disease (IgA, tissue transglutaminase antibodies) is required, particularly if there is a personal or family history of autoimmune conditions.

3. Would your approach be different if she was in the third trimester rather than first?

The World Health Organization definition of anaemia in pregnancy is a haemoglobin less than 110 g/L in the first trimester and less than 105 g/L in the second and third trimesters, which reflects the physiological changes that occur. This patient has a profoundly low haemoglobin which is significantly abnormal irrespective of the trimester in which this is identified. The identification of anaemia at this early gestation makes pregnancy-related causes (e.g. malabsorption due to vomiting, physiological volume expansion in pregnancy) unlikely. Often when anaemia is identified later in pregnancy, empirical oral iron therapy is appropriate with assessment of iron indices if this fails to result in an improvement after a few weeks of therapy. This is not appropriate in this case and urgent assessment is required.

4. What are the potential consequences for the pregnancy?

The presence of maternal anaemia of any cause will exacerbate fatigue in pregnancy, and it is known to increase the incidence of postnatal depression and postpartum haemorrhage. Maternal anaemia has also been associated with increased maternal and neonatal mortality. With respect to the infant, both preterm birth and low birth-weight have been associated with the presence of maternal anaemia. There are also concerns about neonatal neurodevelopment if iron stores are very low.

Iron studies and haematinics are performed, and the results are as follows in Table 55.2:

Table 55.2 Iron studies and haematinics

Serum iron	15 µmol/L
Transferrin	3.9 g/L
Transferrin saturation	8%
Ferritin	10 mcg/L
Folate	7.8 mcg/L
B12	160 ng/L

Questions

5. What conclusion should be made from these results?
6. How would you treat her?
7. Are there any other tests that you would arrange?

Answers

5. What conclusion should be made from these results?

Whilst serum iron is commonly reported when iron studies are performed, it is of no diagnostic use due to great variation during the day. Ferritin is an excellent marker of iron deficiency, although is an acute phase reactant so may be elevated in inflammatory states. An increase in transferrin is seen in iron deficiency. Transferrin saturation is the most specific marker of iron deficiency. The abnormally low ferritin, transferrin saturation, and increased transferrin are therefore all consistent with iron deficiency.

Reassuringly her folate and B12 are within the normal range so her anaemia is not the result of a mixed deficiency picture.

6. How would you treat her?

She requires urgent iron supplementation. *Oral iron* is a reasonable first-line option, and if there is no malabsorption, her haemoglobin should gradually increase over the next few weeks. It is important to advise women of the correct way to take oral iron, on an empty stomach, ideally with orange juice as the ascorbic acid increases iron absorption. Tannins in tea or calcium in dairy products can reduce absorption, so these should not be taken at the same time as the iron supplements. Previously iron supplements were often prescribed 2 or 3 times daily. Recent research shows that absorption is increased when iron supplements are taken less frequently (once daily or on alternate days) because of the effects on hepcidin (oral iron increases hepcidin which in turn reduces gastrointestinal iron absorption). She should be warned about the common gastrointestinal side effects such as nausea and constipation.

Parenteral iron is commonly used in pregnancy, but often avoided in the first trimester. It is a reasonable treatment option later in pregnancy if malabsorption is present, a trial of oral iron has failed to result in an increased haemoglobin, or the woman cannot tolerate oral iron because of the side effects. It is also used if an increase in the haemoglobin is required more quickly than that which would be achieved with oral iron, e.g. if birth is imminent. There have been concerns about anaphylaxis with older iron preparations, but newer preparations such as ferrous carboxymaltose have a very low incidence of anaphylaxis so women can be reassured.

Blood transfusion is rarely required when anaemia has developed gradually, and it is preferable to treat the underlying cause of the anaemia rather than give a transfusion. Very occasionally a blood transfusion is warranted, e.g. if anaemia is so severe that high-output cardiac failure has resulted, or prior to a complex delivery where significant bleeding is likely, e.g. placenta praevia. In this scenario, 1 unit should be transfused followed by clinical assessment to determine whether a further unit is necessary.

7. Are there any other tests that you would arrange?

In iron deficiency it is crucial to establish the cause as described above. Tests for coeliac disease should be performed. If there is no clear cause of the iron deficiency identified, or any symptoms suggestive of gastrointestinal bleeding, then upper and lower gastrointestinal endoscopy is warranted. This can be performed in pregnancy, but decisions about timing should be individualized depending on the exact clinical details.

Further reading

1. UK guidelines on the management of iron deficiency in pregnancy. British Journal of Haematology. 2020; **188**: 819–30. <https://onlinelibrary.wiley.com/doi/epdf/10.1111/bjh.16221>

List of cases by diagnosis

List of cases by principal presentation at diagnosis

List of cases by system

Index